ACUPRESSURE
THERAPY

The characters on the cover mean
'striking point treatment method'
or point percussion therapy, and
are in the author's own
handwriting.

ACUPRESSURE THERAPY

POINT PERCUSSION TREATMENT OF CEREBRAL BIRTH INJURY, BRAIN INJURY AND STROKE

WANG ZHAO-PU MD

Professor

Institute of Orthopaedics and Traumatology

China Academy of Traditional Chinese Medicine,

Beijing

Foreword by
G.C.Schofield OBE MD DPhil FRACP FRACMA
Former Dean of Medicine, Monash University, Melbourne

Churchill Livingstone ▦

MELBOURNE EDINBURGH LONDON
NEW YORK AND TOKYO 1991

CHURCHILL LIVINGSTONE
Medical Division of Longman Group UK Limited

Distributed in Australia by Longman Cheshire Pty Limited, Longman House, Kings Gardens, 95 Coventry Street, South Melbourne 3205, and by associated companies, branches and representatives throughout the world.

First published 1991

ISBN 0-443-04463-5

National Library of Australia Cataloguing in Publication Data

Wang, Zhao-pu.
Acupressure therapy: point percussion treatment of cerebral birth injury, brain injury and stroke.

Bibliography.
Includes index.
ISBN 0 443 04463 5.

1. Acupressure. 2. Brain damage - Patients - Rehabilitation. I. Title.

616.80622

Library of Congress Cataloging-in-Publication Data

Wang, Zhao-pu.
        Acupressure therapy: point percussion treatment of cerebral birth injury, brain injury and stroke / Wang Zhao-pu; foreword by G.C.Schofield.
        p. cm.
    ISBN 0 443 04463 5
    1. Brain damage - Physical therapy. 2. Cerebrovascular disease - Physical therapy.
    3. Birth injuries - Physical therapy. 4. Acupuncture.   I. Title.
        [DNLM: 1. Acupuncture Therapy - methods. 2. Birth injuries - therapy.
    3. Brain Injuries - therapy. 4. Cerebrovascular Disorders - therapy. WS 405 W246a]
    RC387.5.W36   1991
    616.8'04622 - dc20
    DNLM/DLC
    for Library of Congress   .91 - 29426
                                                                         CIP

Produced by Longman Singapore Publishers (Pte) Ltd

Printed in Singapore

FOREWORD

Many forms of medical treatment in both Western and traditional Chinese medicine have their origin in empirical procedures, which through trial and error, have been shown by suitably detached observers to be of benefit to patients. Therapies which alleviate distress or bring ease and comfort to the patient have been retained over the centuries even if the scientific background to their effects has not always been fully understood.

During the period from January to December 1989 Professor Wang Zhao-pu of the Institute of Orthopaedics and Traumatology at the China Academy of Traditional Chinese Medicine in Beijing, together with his assistant, Dr Yu Meng-de, made a visit to Melbourne at the instigation of Ms Jan Bull to begin a programme of treatment for children with cerebral birth injury (cerebral palsy) using a form of treatment which included that described as acupressure therapy. This visit was organized through the Commonwealth Department of Immigration as part of a skills transfer scheme. Professor Wang, who graduated in medicine after studying a conventional undergraduate medical course, practised as an orthopaedic surgeon for some 25 years. He then underwent a period of training in traditional Chinese medicine. Thus he brought with him clinical skills from two medical cultures.

During his stay, Professor Wang completed the major part of this book, in which he describes techniques, methods of assessment, and the outcome of his treatment , for disorders associated with cerebral birth injury, and brain damage following head injury or cerebro-vasular accidents (strokes). Displaying remarkable energy, he wrote at the end of long days. He personally treated the patients, showing now the assured skills of a highly experienced orthopaedic surgeon, including moulding splints into optimal forms, now the careful and confident movements of the physiotherapist, percussing here along stimulation lines and there on pressure points, which perhaps not by chance, covered the geometrical centres of so many muscles, the points at which their nerve supply and major blood supply enters. Sometimes he appeared as a fond grandfather, sometimes as a genial uncle or a family friend; always he was the encouraging counsellor to patients and their families. In his hands Western medicine and traditional Chinese medicine converged on one objective - the recovery of whatever function could be regained - with the understanding that the patient with the assistance of the family should play the major part in that recovery.

Sadly, towards the end of 1989, Professor Wang had an illness which led to a stay in hospital, and after a brief period of recuperation it was judged appropriate for him to return to his home in Beijing. The book was completed during Professor Wang's convalescence.

There are many minor miracles in our everyday life: the ability to perceive movement and colour; to hear sounds and enjoy them; at a younger age to chase after a ball thrown in the air and catch it; to be able at a more advanced

age to walk towards a chosen object without
discomfort; to be able to exercise judgement
and employ intuition (that enigmatic process
we understand so poorly); to engage in a
wide range of other mental, physical and
emotional activities; to enjoy physical effort
and fatigue, and to live without constant
pain; to share the companionship of
congenial people and communicate readily
with them; to have the ability to draw on
thousands of enjoyable or comforting
memories; in short to enjoy good health.

Our perceptions and movements, and our
thoughts and our speech stem from the
activities of many millions of nerve cells
located in the brain and spinal cord. The
organization of these nerve cells into groups
concerned with specific functions follows
genetic instructions built into the original
DNA strands of the single cell, the fertilized
ovum, which is the origin of what later
becomes a human life. That single cell has the
potential to draw on all the qualities of both
parents, except for one genetic decision
already determined by chance that in turn
determines the sex of the future infant.

After cerebral birth injury, significant
though the damage may be, there are large
areas of the brain and many millions of nerve
cells which are still intact. These areas and
the cells they contain are the targets of
education for future living. No child with
cerebral palsy has exactly the same future as
any other with the same condition although
they may share common disabilities. They all
need support, love, affection and
encouragement, if they are to obtain as fully
as possible the share of minor miracles
potentially available to them. They do not

need pity, despair or neglect. They too bring
joy to the family, are proud of achievement
and have their own developmental
milestones, which as for all children are
limitless in number.

During 1989 a visitor from China came to
Australia with a colleague. The visitor met a
group of people who became his friends. In
this book he gives an account of what they
did together. It seems to me that they
achieved a great deal.

G.C.Schofield
Melbourne, 1991

PREFACE

In January 1989, I was invited by the Australia-China Friendship Society to visit Melbourne to lecture on Chinese acupressure therapy and treat patients suffering from the sequelae of cerebral birth injury, brain damage and cerebrovascular accident (CVA).

This book is based on the material used for lectures in Australia, supplemented by many years of teaching and clinical experience, as well as by recent research. The book lays emphasis on the integration of theory with clinical practice. It is in keeping with the great heritage of traditional Chinese medicine in which clinical assessment and manipulative technique go hand in hand. I have also attempted to provide an explanation of the curative mechanism of acupressure therapy in terms of modern science. The book was written at the request of students and published with a view to introducing the method to the Western world. I hope that it will be of benefit to doctors and their patients.

The book consists of six chapters. Chapter 1 is a brief introduction to acupressure therapy. Chapter 2 deals with basic techniques, acupressure points and the stimulation lines for acupressure treatment. It also includes a description of the five basic manipulations in acupressure and methods of examinaton and diagnosis. Chapter 3 discusses the various treatments for specific dysfunctions.

Chapter 4 deals with treatment of cerebral birth injury. In Chapters 5 and 6 the treatment of brain damage and cerebrovascular accident respectively are discussed.

I would like to thank Ms Jill Schofield for helping with my English. I am also greatly indebted to Sarah Dixon, Pamela Fok, Ann Booth, Susan Vincent, Jan Bull, Andre David Menash and Yu Meng-de for their great help in completing this book. My thanks also go to my publisher, Judy Waters, and her staff for preparing my manuscript for publication.

I would sincerely appreciate comments and suggestions from my readers so that I can make improvements in future editions.

Wang Zhao-pu
Beijing, 1991

PUBLISHERS' NOTE

The publishers would like to express thanks for their help in preparing Professor Wang's manuscript for publication to Steven Clavey, Dong Xu-jing, Graeme Schofield, and Yu Meng-de.

CONTENTS

CHAPTER 1

INTRODUCTION

It is not generally known in the West that Chinese medicine, like Western medicine, has a number of specialties and departments. Acupuncture is one of the specialties, and probably the best known, but others include traditional internal medicine, herbal paediatrics, gynaecology, dermatology, geriatrics, orthopaedics, and traumatology. Each has literally centuries of continuing refinement through clinical observation and the accumulation of experience: many of these specialties were established as separate departments in medical colleges as early as the Song dynasty in the thirteenth century. The therapy described in this book is an example of a relatively new technique in traditional Chinese orthopaedics, resulting from a combination of acupuncture theory, martial arts, and traditional orthopaedic manipulation.

Acupuncture theory is based on 'channels' and 'points', the former being a concept of linkages between different areas of the body, the latter being discrete locations along those channels where a stimulus has been found to have a broader effect than one applied, say, at random.

Martial arts (*Wu Shu*) reached a high degree of sophistication in China. In the centuries before the widespread use of guns, the search for even more effective hand-to-hand techniques resulted in a fever of secrecy and experimentation. One of the products was the use of certain acupuncture points struck with great force to numb, immobilize, or even kill an opponent. Although famous to the point of legend in China, the technique itself is not often taught.

Traditional Chinese orthopaedics has probably more similarities to Western medicine than any other department in Chinese medicine, because it deals almost exclusively with the structure of the body rather than its internal functioning. Very briefly, the main differences are fourfold:

1. Western orthopaedics tends to focus on the treatment of bones, while Chinese orthopaedics places equal emphasis on bones and the fibrous or soft tissues associated with them.

2. Chinese orthopaedic techniques are similar to the Western techniques, but the range and variety is greater. This is another product of the race for martial arts 'technology' mentioned above: increased experimentation with hand-to-hand techniques (many involving joint twisting or deliberate dislocation) naturally resulted in increased injuries, and consequently methods of treatment were developed to deal with them. This is why the full name of this specialty is, in China, 'Orthopaedics and Traumatology'.

3. Chinese orthopaedics utilizes the acupuncture channel and point theory in conjunction with standard orthopaedic technique, and will use acupuncture itself, or acupressure, or massage along the channels, or moxibustion (stimulation of acupuncture points by heat) to achieve the stated aim of all Chinese medical

interventions: 'harmonious functioning and unobstructed interaction'.

4. Chinese herbs will also be used, in a variety of forms such as decoctions or pills taken internally, plasters, soaks, compresses, or poultices applied externally, and herbs intended to speed the knitting of bones held within a soft changeable cast.

The three factors of acupuncture theory, martial arts, and traditional orthopaedic manipulation combined in 1983. I led a team from the Institute of Orthopaedics and Traumatology in Beijing, to Shandong province, to investigate claims that the ancient martial arts technique had been adapted effectively for the treatment of diseases such as sequelae of poliomyelitis or CVA, paraplegia, lumbago, and so on. We discovered that this was in fact the case, after observing the treatments of Mr Jia Li-hui, who had developed the technique based on the martial arts point-striking technology and certain breathing exercises, both of which had been passed down through his family. He had been using point percussion therapy since the 1960s, and had established an acupressure department at the Laoshan county hospital in Shandong province. After assessing the results of the treatments on a sample of 65 patients, the decision was made to introduce the technique into clinical practice at the Beijing Institute of Orthopaedics and Traumatology.

CHINESE MEDICINE

For centuries Chinese medicine has gathered clinical experience, all described in the same stringently defined terms, and therefore accessible to a modern practitioner of traditional Chinese medicine. It is this incredible wealth of medical experience that is one of the strengths of Chinese medicine and was described by Mao Ze-dong as 'a vast treasure-house'.

The theoretical system itself is relatively simple, and practical for the clinic, with a minimum of technical aids, and is based primarily upon the combination of the patient's subjective impressions and the physician's own observations and examinations. Now this, of course, would be exactly the same as Western clinical diagnosis, except that:

1. The fundamental theory draws the attention of the Chinese doctor to a different set of clinical patterns (both symptomatic and syndromatic) from those of Western medicine.

2. Greater emphasis is placed on the context of the individual symptom, so that the subjective impressions of the patient receive a higher priority in Chinese medicine than in Western medicine.

Several striking differences of approach between the two medicines must be mentioned, though. The first is that Chinese medicine has maintained a concept of 'strengthening' the patient, which receives as much attention as 'attacking' the perceived cause of a problem. (This has been found in China to be a useful area of cooperation between the two medicines, e.g., in cancer therapy where Chinese herbs are used to support the patient during chemo- or radio-therapy, and reduce the side effects of these 'attacks'.)

The second difference in approach is the general concept within Chinese medicine of 'harmonious functioning and uninterrupted interaction', between the various parts of the body. This is similar to the Western 'homeostasis' concept except that 'stasis' is completely foreign to the Chinese idea of health. All is in constant flux and change, from the most ethereal mental processes (the 'Spirit'), to the somewhat more material breath moving in and out of the lungs, to the still visibly altering flesh and muscle, down to the deepest, slowest level of change, the bones.

Each part of a person's body is seen to be not only related and linked to, but a reflection of, every other part. Therefore pain or tissue changes in certain areas will lead the Chinese doctor to consider pathology in organs related by either acupuncture channel or natural affinity (e.g., heart and blood vessels).

The last great difference in approach concerns the 'level' of diagnosis in Chinese medicine. Chinese diagnostics does not work at the level of cellular pathology, but rather at the level of functional disruption of the organism as a whole. It is based on the patient's perceptions of discomfort, plus the physician's careful (yet technologically unaided) examination, although Chinese treatment based on Western diagnosis (e.g., X-ray) is not uncommon.

As these strengths and weaknesses of the two medicines became appreciated in China, the advantages of cooperation and a combined two-stream system also became obvious. Over the last 30 years or so such a system has been operating not only in China, but also in Japan.

THEORETICAL ASPECTS OF ACUPRESSURE

Acupressure is based on the same theory as acupuncture and uses the same points and meridians. The meridians are the key to the human body's ability to adapt to its surroundings. If the normal functions of the meridians are disturbed by pathogenic factors such as infection, trauma, Cold, Heat, Damp, etc., disease will occur. The therapeutic effect of acupressure technique lies in the way in which it regulates and normalizes the blocked functions of the meridians. In traditional Chinese medicine the meridians are considered to be the channels of Vital Energy *(Qi)* with the function of harmonizing Yin and Yang, and nourishing the Organs, muscles and bones of the human body. The Blood, Yin and Yang, and muscles and bones are in turn controlled by the meridians. The meridians are the key means by which the balance between the Interior and Exterior, the Yin and Yang, of the body is maintained.

In the light of our clinical experience and laboratory research at the Institute of Orthopaedics and Traumatology the therapeutic effect of acupressure may be summarized as follows:

1. Regulating the balance of Yin and Yang

2. Clearing the meridians and stimulating the circulation of Blood and Vital Energy

3. Improving the conductivity of the nerves

4. Bringing about an improvement in the general condition of patients.

Regulating the balance of Yin and Yang

The relationship between Yin and Yang is close and continuous. Yin and Yang are the two fundamental attributes in the universe always complementing and opposing each other - an ancient philosophical idea used in traditional Chinese medicine to conceptualize various dualities in anatomy, physiology, pathology, diagnosis and clinical treatment. By the grand harmony of Yin and Yang good health is guaranteed.

Yin is the negative principle, the material or structural aspect of things. Feminine, interior, cold and hypofunction are Yin. Yin disorders are due in general to some deficiency of Vital Function or the body's resistance.

Yang is the positive principle, the active or functional aspect of things. Masculine, exterior, heat, and hyperfunction are Yang. Yang disorders are due to an excess of Heat or activity resulting from an exogenous pathogenic factor or internal imbalance.

If the balance of Yin and Yang is disturbed, resulting in too much of one and too little of the other, disease will occur. The Vital Energy (life depends upon Vital Energy (*Qi*)) that circulates in the meridians will be obstructed. If the blockage is removed by means of acupressure, the Vital Energy will again circulate normally along the meridians, the balance between Yin and Yang will be restored, and the patient will recover.

In the patients at our clinic with sequelae of cerebral birth injury, brain injury and cerebrovascular accidents, 87% of cases showed spastic manifestations. This is a disorder of excess Yang and lack of Yin in those patients. Acupressure manipulations brought relief to these patients after 60 to 70 sessions of treatment by decreasing the spasticity of the affected muscles.

On the other hand, we had 13% of patients with weakness of the muscles. The preponderance of Yin impairs Yang. Yin disease is a deficiency disorder with lowered Vital Function and weak muscles. These patients also received acupressure therapy. We found that, after 60 to 70 sessions of treatment, the previously weak muscle tone increased.

Acupressure can regulate the balance of Yin and Yang. Thus the therapy can both decrease the spasticity of affected muscles and increase the muscle tone of weak muscles. This is the most important effect of the method in the treatment of cerebral palsy.

Clearing the meridians and stimulating smooth circulation of Blood and Vital Energy

When disease is present, the pathogenic factors causing the disease will interfere with the body's own normal mechanisms, and the meridians become blocked, so that the circulation of Vital Energy and Blood circulation are obstructed. Acupressure therapy can support and strengthen the healthy energy, expel the pathogenic factors, and lead to a smooth blood circulation so that the disease is reversed.

The purpose of this book is to provide an account of acupressure therapy, its background, and the outcome of its application to a self-selected group of patients. It is not intended to attempt to describe in any detail our previous clinical and laboratory research. This includes research involving animal models, which examines basic biological mechanisms involved in and underlying the therapeutic process. It relates, for example, to improvement in the blood circulation and nerve conductivity with consequent improvement in muscle function. The biological background to these gains, is generally well understood in clinical and scientific communities as is appropriate education or re-education for voluntary movement in unused or wasted muscles leading to correction of limb deformity.

Further, the results of our own studies support the view that acupressure therapy is accompanied by a lowering of arterial diastolic blood pressure, without change to heart rate, systolic pressure or stroke volume. It suggests that there is decreased peripheral resistance in arterioles and improved peripheral blood circulation, which was confirmed by studies on microcirculation in human nail folds and pial vessels in experimental animals. Research was carried out on the cerebral haemodynamics of patients with cerebral birth injury before and after acupressure therapy. Scanning techniques were used in monitoring the passage of short half-life radioactive materials through the cerebral circulation; in almost one-third of the patients the regional cerebral blood flow was increased after acupressure therapy ranging from 28-60 sessions.

Other studies involved sampling blood from dogs before and after acupressure procedures, which were carried out for 20 minutes. These studies showed that the viscosity of plasma and whole blood, the adhesiveness of blood platelets, and the content of fibrinogen were all lowered to statistically significant levels. Little change was found in either the sedimentation rate of red blood cells or the blood cell volume.

In clinical practice, after a period of acupressure treatment, the patients feel a general ease, sleep soundly, have more energy, a good appetite and appear to have better resistance to disease.

The advantages of acupressure therapy are that some main deformities can be corrected and that joint functions can be restored to the normal or near normal range. It is essential, however, that an appropriate set of exercises through a full range of movement at affected joints is continued after acupressure therapy if progressive therapeutic gains so essential to the recovery of such patients are to be made.

CHAPTER 2
TECHNIQUES AND ASSESSMENT

Acupressure modifies the forceful movements of *Wu Shu* (martial arts) to a degree that is not too hard upon the normal human body. The therapy is applied with the fingers on the points and the stimulation lines of the body surface. Although there is some similarity between acupressure and acupuncture, the mode of action of acupressure is quite different from that of acupuncture: the manipulative technique is simple, there is no need for drugs or special instruments, and acupressure can be coped with easily by patients. It is safe and effective in clinical practice.

POINTS FOR ACUPRESSURE THERAPY

About 120 points selected from those used in acupuncture and the martial arts are employed in the therapy described in this book. The points are listed on pages 12 and 13. Their location is shown schematically in Figures 2.1, 2.2 and 2.3. Descriptions of the location of specific points are given throughout the book. Please note that any measurements given in these descriptions are for adults.

Acupressure points

• Points on the head and neck

Baihui, DU 20 百會

Shuaigu, G8 率谷

Naokong, G19 腦空

Bige, MA point 鼻隔

Yuyao, Extra 3 魚腰

Wangu, G12 完骨

Chengqi, S1 承泣

Sibai, S2 四白

Jingming, B1 睛明

Yamen, DU15 啞門

Dicang, S4 地倉

Chengjiang, Ren 24 承漿

Yingxiang, LI 20 迎香

Lianquan, Ren 23 廉泉

Jiachengjiang, Extra 5 夾承漿

Sizhukong, SJ 23 絲竹空

Tinggong, SI 19 聽宮

Tinghui, G2 聽會

Chuigen, MA point 垂根

Fengchi, G20 風池

Tianzhu B10 天柱

Suliao, DU 25 素膠

Dazhui, DU 14 大椎

Taiyang, Extra 2 太陽

Touwei, S8 頭維

Zengyin, Extra 11 增音

Yifeng, SJ 17 翳風

• Points on the thoracic and abdominal wall

Tiantu, Ren 22 天突

Quepen, S12 缺盆

Shanzhong, Ren 17 膻中

Jiuwei, Ren 15 鳩尾

Shangwan, Ren 13 上脘

Zhongwan, Ren 12 中脘

Qihai, Ren 6 氣海

Guanyuan, Ren 4 關元

Zhongji, Ren 3 中極

Qichong, S30 氣冲

Qugu, Ren 2 曲骨

Huiyin, Ren 1 會陰

• Points on the back and lumbar region

Jianjing, G21 肩井

Bingfeng, SI12 秉風

Tianzong, SI11 天宗

Jianzhen, SI 9 肩貞

Fufen, B41 附分

Fengmen, B12 風門

Geshu, B17 膈俞

Yaoyan, Extra 37 腰眼

Guanyuanshu B26 關元俞

Pangguanshu, B28 膀胱俞

•**Points on the upper limb**

Jianyu, LI 15　肩髃

Tianquan, P2　天泉

Binao, LI 14　臂臑

Naohui, SJ 13　臑會

Zhima, MA point　肢麻

Quchi, LI 11　曲池

Jihui, MA point　肌滙

Ximen, P4　郄門

Neiguan, P6　內關

Daling, P7　大陵

Sidu, SJ 9　四瀆

Waiguan, SJ 5　外關

Jianshi, P5　間使

Xiabai, LU 4　俠白

Yangxi, LI 5　陽溪

Yangchi, SJ 4　陽池

Hegu, LI 4　合谷

Zhangjian, MA point　掌間

Zhiguanjie, MA point　指關節

Zhijiagen, MA point　指甲根

• **Points on the lower limb**

Huantiao, G30　環跳

Chengfu, B36　承扶

Yinmen, B37　殷門

Weizhong, B40　委中

Fuxi, B38　浮郄

Chengshan, B57　承山

Genjian, MA point　跟腱

Biguan S31　髀關

Futu, S32　伏兔

Heding, Extra 31　鶴頂

Fenglong, S40　豐隆

Jiexi, S41　解溪

Zusanli, S36　足三里

Fengshi, G31　風市

Yinlingquan, SP 9　陰陵泉

Yanglingquan, G34　陽陵泉

Jimen, SP 11　箕門

Lougu, SP 7　漏谷

Xiehai, SP 10　血海

Taichong, Liv 3　太冲

Zulinqi G41　足臨泣

Yongquan, K1　湧泉

Zhijiagen, MA point　趾甲根

Zhiguanjie, MA point　趾關節

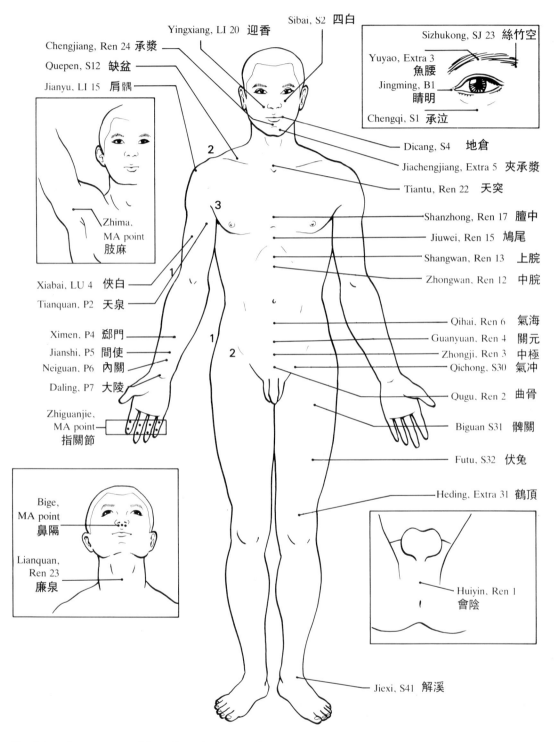

Fig. 2.1   Acupressure points on the anterior aspect

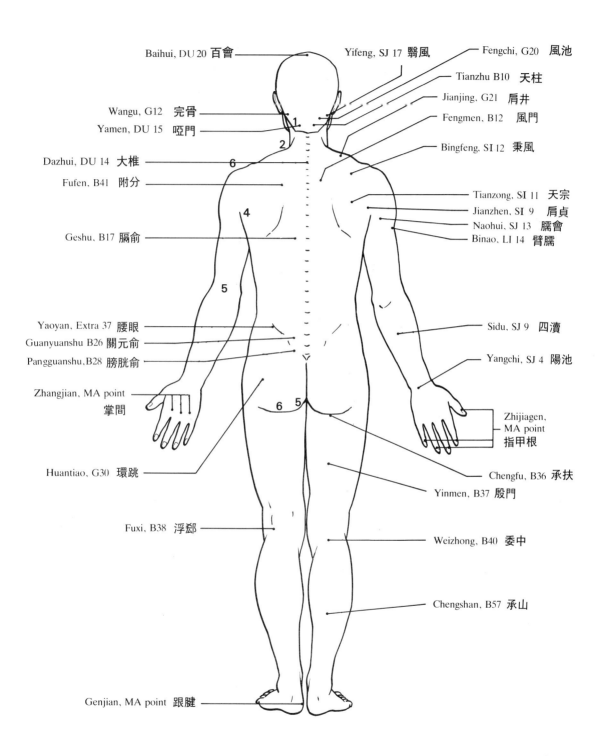

Fig. 2.2 Acupressure points on the posterior aspect

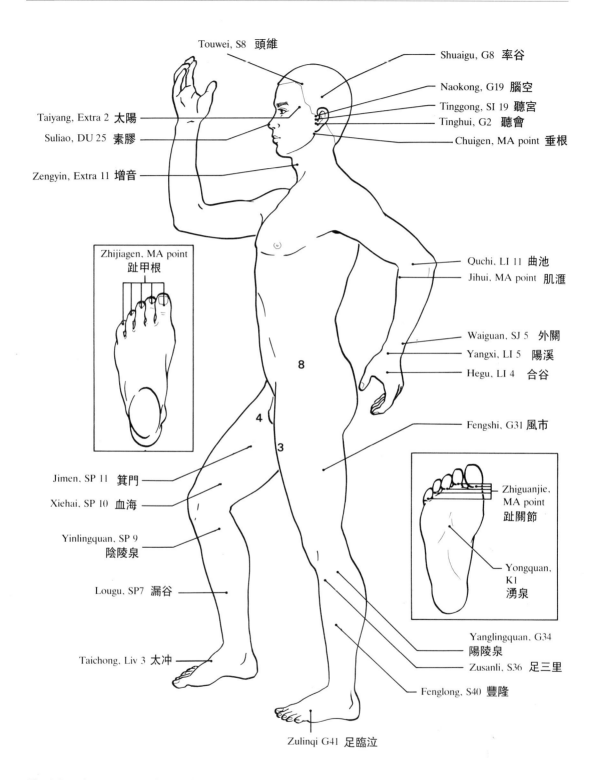

Fig. 2.3 Acupressure points on the lateral aspect

STIMULATION LINES

There are sixteen stimulation lines distributed on the body surface. Their location is shown schematically in Figures 2.4, 2.5 and 2.6.

Stimulation lines

• Lines on the upper limb

There are 6 lines (see Figs 2.4 and 2.5).

The first line
This extends from the lateral end of the flexion crease of the wrist upward along the radial side of the forearm through the prominence of the Brachioradialis muscle to finish at the lateral end of the flexion crease of the elbow joint. It corresponds to part of the hand Taiyin lung meridian (手太陰肺徑).

The second line
This extends from the mid-point of the flexion crease of the wrist , proceeds upward along the mid-line of the forearm and arm to the anterior part of the shoulder joint. It corresponds to part of the hand Jueyin peri-cardium meridian (手厥陰心包徑).

The third line
This extends from the medial end of the flexion crease of the wrist, proceeds upward along the medial side of the forearm and arm to the anterior end of the axillary line. It corresponds to part of the hand Shaoyin heart meridian (手少陰心徑).

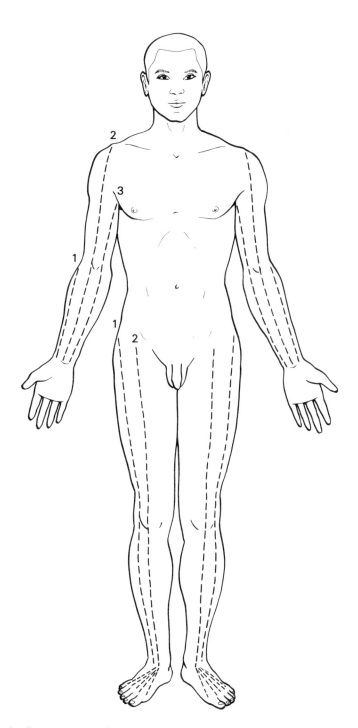

Fig. 2.4 Stimulation lines on the anterior aspect

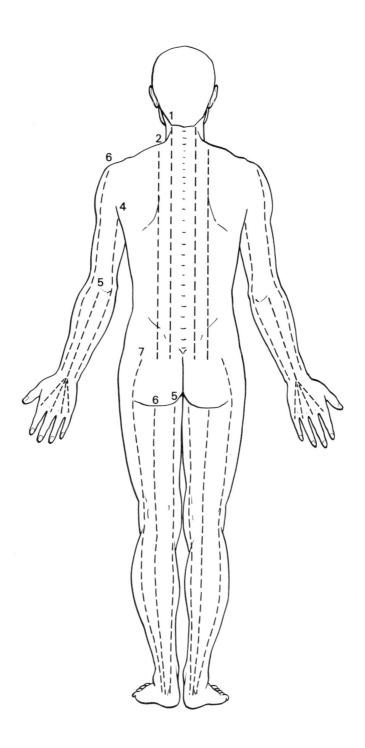

Fig. 2.5 Stimulation lines on the posterior aspect

• **Lines on the upper limb cont.**

The fourth line
This extends from the medial end of the extension creases of the wrist upward along the medial side of the forearm and arm to the posterior end of the axillary line. It corresponds to part of the hand Taiyang small intestine meridian (手太陽小腸徑).

The fifth line
This converging line extends from the dorsal aspect of the medial four metacarpophalangeal joints, and proceeds upward along each tendon of Extensor digitorum muscle. The lines join on the dorsal aspect of the wrist. It then proceeds upward as a single line along the mid-line of the dorsal aspect of the forearm, as far as the elbow joint. It corresponds to part of the Sanjiao meridian of the hand Shaoyang (手太陽三焦徑).

The sixth line
This extends from the lateral end of the extension creases of the wrist upward along the lateral side of the forearm and arm as far as the acromion. It corresponds to part of the hand Yangming large intestine meridian (手陽明大腸徑).

• **Lines on the back and lumbar region**
There are two double lines (see Fig. 2.5).

The first line
This first pair extends from the posterior hair margin downward 5 cm lateral to the spinal column on each side as far as the lumbosacral joint. The double line corresponds to part of the first line on the back of the foot Taiyang bladder meridian (足太陽膀胱徑).

The second line
This second pair extends from each side of the first thoracic vertebra downward 8 cm lateral to the spinal column on both as far as the sacrum. The line corresponds to part of the second line on the back of the foot Taiyang bladder meridian (足太陽膀胱徑).

- **Lines on the lower limb**
There are 8 lines (see Figs 2.4, 2.5, and 2.6).

The first line
This starts anterior to the ankle joint, ascends first in front of the Tibialis anterior muscle, then lateral to the patella then ascends on the lateral surface of the thigh to reach the iliac crest posterior to the anterior superior iliac spine. It corresponds to part of the foot Yangming stomach meridian (足陽明胃徑).

The second line
These converging lines start from the dorsal aspect of the five metatarsophalangeal joints of the foot and follow the tendons of the Extensor digitorum longus muscle to a point anterior to the ankle joint. Here the lines unite and ascend as a single line through the lateral aspect of, in turn, the Tibialis anterior muscle, the lateral side of the knee joint and the thigh, to reach the anterior superior iliac spine. It corresponds to part of the foot Shaoyang gall bladder meridian (足少陽膽徑).

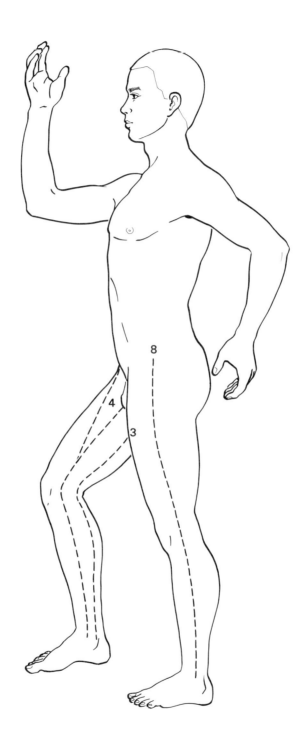

Fig. 2.6 Stimulation lines on the lower limbs

- **Lines on the lower limb cont.**

The third line

This starts from the medial side of the Tendo calcaneus (Achilles tendon), and proceeds upward along the medial side of the Gastrocnemius muscle, the knee joint, and the Gracilis muscle terminating at its upper attachment. It corresponds to part of the foot Shaoyin kidney meridian (足少陰腎徑).

The fourth line

This starts from the posterior fossa of the medial malleolus, and ascends on the leg to the medial side of the knee joint, where it divides into two branches: one branch follows the Sartorius muscle to the anterior superior iliac spine; the other branch follows the medial margin of the Adductor magnus muscle, and terminates in the region of the superficial inguinal ring. This line corresponds to parts of the foot Jueyin liver meridian (足厥陰肝徑之一部), and the foot Taiyin spleen meridian (足太陰脾徑之一部).

The fifth line

This starts from the insertion of the Tendo calcaneus (Achilles tendon), ascends along the posteromedial aspect of the leg and thigh to reach the ischial tuberosity. It corresponds to part of the foot Taiyang bladder meridian (足太陽膀胱徑之一部分).

The sixth line

This starts from the mid-point of the insertion of the Tendo calcaneus, and ascends vertically to the mid-point of the popliteal fossa and then the ischial tuberosity. It corresponds to part of the foot Taiyang bladder meridian (足太陽膀胱徑之一部分).

• **Lines on the lower limb cont.**

The seventh line
This starts from the lateral malleolus, and ascends along the lateral margin of the Gastrocnemius muscle and then lateral to the popliteal fossa, and Biceps femoris muscle, before passing over the greater trochanter of the femur to reach the posterior superior iliac spine.

The eighth line
This starts from the lateral malleolus, proceeds upward along the prominence of the Peroneus longus muscle to reach the head of the fibula, and the lateral margin of the patella and then ascends along the Vastus lateralis muscle to reach the summit of the iliac crest. It corresponds to part of the foot Shaoyang gall bladder meridian (足少陽膽徑之一部分).

FIVE BASIC MANIPULATIONS

Acupressure therapy is administered using the basic techniques or 'manipulations', which I have described over the page.

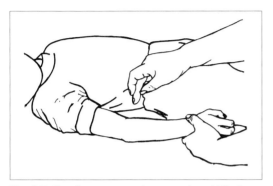

Fig. 2.7 One finger percussion uses the middle finger braced by the thumb and index finger

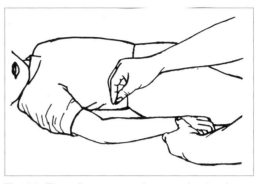

Fig. 2.8 Three finger percussion uses the thumb, index and middle fingers

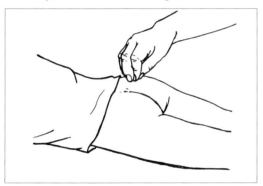

Fig. 2.9 Five finger percussion uses the thumb and all four fingers

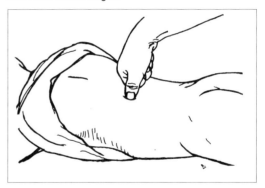

Fig. 2.10 First form of pressing: the four fingers are bent with the thumb extended

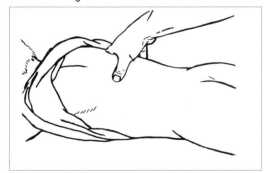

Fig. 2.11 Second form of pressing: hold the area under treatment with the thumb on one side and the four fingers on the opposite side. The thumb is moved up, down right and left, and round and round, but should not slide on or rub the skin

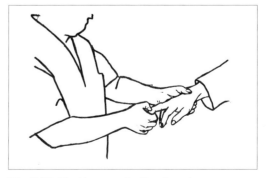

Fig. 2.12 Pinching: use the thumb and index finger to pinch on the nailfold, or any part of the thumb and fingers, or the foot

Basic Manipulations

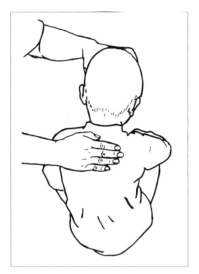

Fig. 2.13 Clapping: clap with the palm of the hand to relieve the reaction to manipulation or to relax spasm of the muscles. This is usually applied to the head or back of the patient

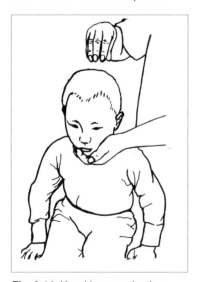

Fig. 2.14 Knocking: use the tips of the fingers for strong stimulation and pads for light stimulation. This is applied on the head and any part of the body

1. Percussion

This is an important and fundamental manipulation of acupressure therapy, and depending on the manoeuvre to be carried out is divided into three types: one finger percussion; three finger percussion; and five finger percussion (see Figs 2.7, 2.8 and 2.9).

Percussion is also divided into three types according to the degree of force applied:

a. Light percussion. This is a movement of the hand from the wrist joint.
b. Medium percussion. This is a movement of the elbow joint, using the force of the fore arm. The wrist joint is fixed or semifixed.
c. Strong percussion. This is a movement of the shoulder joint, using the force of the upper arm. The wrist is fixed.

2. Pressing

This manipulation is done with the thumb. There are two forms of pressing (see Figs 2.10 and 2.11).

3. Pinching

This manipulation involves a normal pinching movement, but is only used on the hands (see Fig. 2.12).

4. Clapping

This manipulation involves striking with the flat of the hand using medium force only (see Fig. 2.13).

5. Knocking

This manipulation differs from percussion in that the hand is loose and the fingers are not grouped together (see Fig. 2.14).

ASSESSMENT PROCEDURES

I have described the procedures for the assessment of patients for their suitability for this form of treatment in relation to children suffering from the sequelae of cerebral birth injury, however the principles of obtaining a full case history, observation of normal daily activities, and clinical examination are relevant to adult patients.

Practitioners involved in acupressure therapy should be familiar with the techniques of physical examination, have a good knowledge of the relevant reflex reactions of children, and ensure that a comprehensive case history is available.

• **Background information**

The case history should include the following:

1. A history and discharge summary from the hospital where the child was delivered.

2. Reports from the doctors, paediatricians and other therapists from whom the child has received treatment since being discharged from hospital.

3. A comprehensive written report from the parent/s relating the case history as they understand it and giving a personal account of any previous or current programme of therapy, of the child's development and behaviour in and out of the home, and of any perceived progress made by the child since being discharged from hospital.

On the basis of the information supplied, the practitioner determines the suitability of the child to begin a programme of acupressure therapy. If the child is considered suitable for therapy, a clinical examination is arranged for later, and further information is sought at that time.

Initial approach to assessment

1. First observe the child in his or her spontaneous behaviour, at home, in the school room or in the playground. Spontaneous behaviour in cerebral palsy children is quite limited, and a child does not usually reveal the potential for a motor ability unless the therapy assessment is specially structured to make him or her do so.

2. In the therapy room, talk to the child's mother first, while you observe the child at play with toys. When the mother accepts you, you will find it easier to assess the child. Also ask the child to bring a favourite toy.

3. There should never be an atmosphere of a 'test' or 'examination' with young children. Much can be obtained during play with the child in familiar surroundings at home or school.

4. Do not undress the child until it feels comfortable and relaxed to do so. Watching him or her undress will offer an excellent opportunity for assessment of features such as posture-balance and hand function.

5. Observations are ongoing so that assessment continues during the course of the therapy.

6. The practitioner may sometimes begin assessment of main functions, for example, the form of locomotion, and the ability to sit, stand or walk, and to rise from a chair, couch, or bed, and may then plan some therapy techniques for these functions. Assessment is continued alongside therapy in the following sessions.

Treatment should be appropriate for the stage of development already reached by the child as this helps obtain his or her co-operation. The practitioner can assess development during therapy and plan the treatment accordingly.

Clinical examinaton

The clinical examination includes all the items on the clinical examination sheet which are relevant to the child (see Fig. 2.15). Clinical findings before and after treatment are recorded.

Typical notations of clinical findings

```
     (++)  normal
      (+)  less than normal
    (+++)  more than normal
    (-ve)  negative finding
           (normal or recovery)
    (+ve)  positive finding
        L  left side
        R  right side
        B  both sides
        A  Absent
       WS  stands for with support
 Number %  percentage may be added.
```

Clinical Examination

Patient's name _____ Chart No _____

Date of birth _____ Name of Institution _____

Date of onset _____ Name of parents _____

Address _____

_____

Telephone _____

DIAGNOSIS

	BEFORE TREATMENT	AFTER TREATMENT		
		Recovery	Improvement	No Change
Mental retardation				
Aprhenia				
Aphasia				
Aphonia				
Dysphasia				
Cerebellar ataxia				
Vision disturbance L R				
Bed-wetting				
Drooling				
Opisthotonus				
Elevation of arm L R				
Brush forehead with upper part of forearm L R				
Touch opposite auricle L R				
Touch spine with thumb L R				
Supination forearm L R				
Drop wrist L R				
Thumb abduction L R				
Clawfinger L R				
Difficulty in grasping L R				
Inability to grasp L R				
Inability to sit				
Inability to stand				
Inability to walk				
Scissor legs				
Limp & sluggish gait L R				

Fig. 2.15 Clinical examination form

DIAGNOSIS Cont.

	BEFORE TREATMENT	AFTER TREATMENT		
		Recovery	Improvement	No Change
Expand hip joint (Frog test)				
Internal rotation of thigh L R				
External rotation of thigh L R				
Stretch & elevation of leg L R				
4-form test in prone position L R				
Contraction iliotibial tract L R				
Allis' sign				
Flexion of knee L R				
Drop foot L R				
Equinovarus L R				
Equinovalgus L R				
Talipes calcaneus L R				
Reflex of tendon biceps brachii L R				
Reflex of tendon triceps brachii L R				
Periosteoradial reflex L R				
Hoffman's sign L R				
Knee jerk reflex				
Reflex Achilles tendon L R				
Babinski's sign L R				
Patellar clonus L R				
Ankle clonus L R				
Abdominal reflex				
Cremasteric reflex L R				
Anal reflex				

Practitioner _____ Date of examination _____

Fig. 2.15 Clinical examination form cont.

Matters for attention in clinical practice

1. First write a case history, then make a diagnosis and plan treatment based on an overall analysis of the illness and the patient's condition, and select points and stimulation lines for the individual patient.

2. Start the manipulations gently and gradually increase the magnitude. Special care should be taken to avoid injury of joint capsules, rupture of tendons and fractures.

3. Patients usually have sensations such as soreness, numbness, warmth and distension in the area of manipulation. A skin flush may occur. Sometimes the patients may sweat or develop a fever. Subcutaneous bleeding may occur at the beginning of treatment, and disappear within a week. None of these reactions needs any special treatment. In case of severe reactions such as dizziness, nausea, paleness of the face or shock, manipulation should be stopped and relaxing measures should be taken immediately. The practitioner may clap the patient on the head and back, and press on the martial art point Bige when necessary. Some patients may feel worse after manipulations in the beginning. This will improve after 3 to 5 days.

4. No food or drink should be taken before or during manipulation. This can be dangerous if the child begins crying and food is inhaled into the bronchi.

5. Where the disability of the patient is pronounced in patients older than 10 years of age (but not including adults with cerebral trauma) and in patients who are not able to receive regular treatment, the results of treatment may be unsatisfactory.

Continuing treatment and care

It is assumed that parents of children with cerebral palsy will involve themselves in carrying on the treatment and the exercises recommended by the practitioner. There is no guarantee as to the curative effect of the treatment, but there are usually obvious signs of improvement after 3 months of continuous treatment.

Frequency and course of treatment

The manipulation may be carried out in sessions once daily, every other day, or every 3 days, according to the condition of the patient. The length of the course of treatment is 20 sessions. A patient may receive treatment of 2 to 3 courses consecutively. However, if the curative effect becomes slow, it is better to stop treatment for a period of up to a month.

 # CONTRAINDICATIONS

The contraindications for acupressure treatment are as follows:

1. Acute diseases, for example, infections, acute abdomen, suppurative arthritis
2. Severe heart disease, tuberculosis, malignant tumours
3. Haemorrhagic diseases, for example, haemophilia, purpura haemorrhagica, haemorrhagic glaucoma, haemorrhagic anaemia
4. Severe skin diseases
5. Poor general condition, for example, malnutrition, asthenia, collapse.

CHAPTER 3

TREATMENTS FOR SPECIFIC DYSFUNCTIONS

This chapter discusses the dysfunctions that are common to cases of cerebral birth injury, brain injury and cerebrovascular accidents, and outlines the methods and techniques used in acupressure therapy to treat them. Included are movement difficulties in the arms, hands and legs, problems with speech and vision, facial paralysis, drooling, difficulty in swallowing and aphagia, and problems of sitting. Although the discussion is linked mainly to cerebral birth injury, procedures for use in all cases are presented.

SOME TERMS OF REFERENCE

In describing deformities and motor disabilities and their treatment, it is necessary to stipulate a standard position of the body and its parts, *the anatomical position of reference*. This allows uniformity in describing movements at joints irrespective of whether the patient is standing upright, or lying in a horizontal position facing upwards (the supine position) or downwards

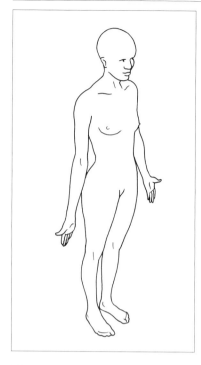

Fig. 3.1 The anatomical position of reference. Reproduced with permission from Chandler J 1991 Tabbner's nursing care: theory and practice, 2nd edition. Churchill Livingstone, Melbourne

(the prone position). In the standard reference position the person is visualized as standing erect with the feet together, the head and eyes directed forwards, and the upper limbs at the side of the body with the palms of the hands directed forwards (see Fig. 3.1).

Movement of the upper limb away from the midline of the body is referred to as *abduction* and its return to the position of reference is *adduction* (this movement occurs at the shoulder joint between the arm and the trunk (see Fig. 3.2A & B)). The same terms are used for similar movements at the wrist joint between the forearm and hand, and at the hip joint between the trunk and the lower limbs.

Forward and backward movements occurring at the shoulder, elbow, and wrist joints ,at the joints of the hand (but not the thumb), and at the hip joints are known as *flexion* and *extension* respectively (see Fig. 3.2C & D).

In mobile joints such as the shoulder, wrist, and hip joints, and joints within the hand and foot rotational movements occur. If the hand is turned (rotated) so that it faces backwards the movement is referred to as *pronation*; a return to the position of reference is referred to as *supination* (see Fig. 3.2H & I).

Different muscles or groups of muscles are involved in producing the movements described and are often, but not always, given names which indicate their function. Thus, there are flexor muscles, extensor muscles, adduction and abduction muscles which are named according to their function. For example, Flexor carpi radialis is a muscle which arises from the lower part of the humerus (the bone of the arm) and is inserted into two of the carpal bones of the hand; it crosses both the elbow and wrist joints, and when it contracts to shorten itself, it leads to flexion movements at both

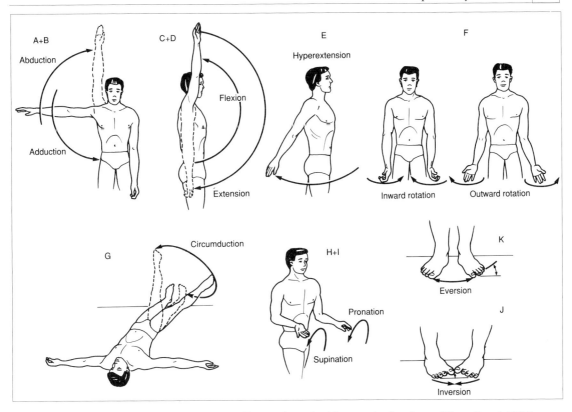

Fig. 3.2 The range of joint movements. Reproduced with permission from Chandler J 1991 Tabbner's nursing care: theory and practice, 2nd edition. Churchill Livingstone, Melbourne

joints. Some muscles are given names for reasons other than to identify their function. For example, the muscle which produces movement of flexion at two joints corresponding to that of Flexor carpi radialis, but in this case at the shoulder and elbow joints, could be named Flexor brachii (the flexion of the upper arm). However this muscle has two heads of origin, from the shoulder blade or scapula, and is known as the two-headed muscle of the arm (Biceps brachii). Its counterpart, which causes extension at the corresponding joints, has three heads of origin and is known as Triceps brachii.

In describing movement of the limbs a number of additional points need to be made. First, the movement of flexion at the knee joint as in kneeling is a backward movement of the leg towards the thigh, and is thus opposite to the corresponding movement of flexion at the elbow joint. Secondly, in the human hand, the thumb is rotated so that the nail of the thumb is at right angles to the plane of the nails of the fingers. Flexion of the thumb leads to it moving towards the midline across the palm, and extension corresponds to a movement of the thumb away from the index finger.

Abduction and adduction occur in the same plane as flexion and extension occurring in the fingers. Finally, at the ankle joint the term *plantar flexion* is used for movements at the ankle joints associated with standing on toes and the term *dorsiflexion* for the movement associated with standing on heels.

General readers should also note that some terms are employed in anatomy in a different sense from everyday usage. For example, *arm* refers to the upper limb between the shoulder and elbow, and *leg* to the lower limb between the knee and ankle.

DEFORMITIES AND DYSFUNCTION OF THE UPPER LIMBS

PROBLEMS OF THE SHOULDER

Shoulder movements

The shoulder joint is composed of the head of the humerus and the glenoid fossa of the scapula. It is a multiaxial joint. The articular capsule is very loose, reinforced in the upper part by the coraco-acromial ligament. Anteriorly, the tendon of the long head of the Biceps muscle passes through the joint, and posteriorly the tendons of the Supra- and Infraspinatus muscles strengthen the shoulder capsule. Looseness of the capsule on the inferior part of the joint often leads to dislocation of the shoulder joint in this position.

Shoulder movements include adduction, abduction, flexion, extension, and internal and external rotations. The muscles involved in movement of the shoulder joint are listed in Table 3.1.

Functional disturbance of movements of the shoulder joint occurs commonly in patients with cerebral birth injury. For the purposes of assessment and treatment we have classified the movements of the shoulder joint into four groups, which are described on page 41.

Table 3.1 Movements of the shoulder joint, the muscles producing the movements, and their nerve supply

Muscle	Nerve supply	Nerve roots
Adduction		
Infraspinatus	Suprascapular nerve	C5, 6
Teres minor	Axillary nerve	C5, 6
Teres major	Lower subscapular nerve	C5,
Subscapularis	Upper and lower subscapular nerve	C5, 6
Latissimus dorsi	Thoracodorsal nerve	C6 - C8
Pectoralis major	Medial and lateral pectoral nerves	C5 - T1
Coracobrachialis	Musculocutaneus nerve	C5 - C7
Internal rotation		
Infrascapularis	Suprascapular nerve	C5, 6
Pectoralis major	Medial and lateral pectoral nerves	C5 - T1
Latissimus dorsi	Thoracodorsal nerve	C6 - C8
Abduction		
Deltoid	Axillary nerve	C5, 6
Supraspinatus	Suprascapular nerve	C5
External rotation		
Infraspinatus	Suprascapular nerve	C5, 6
Teres minor	Axillary nerve	C5, 6
Extension		
Teres major	Lower subscapular nerve	C5, 6
Latissimus dorsi	Thoracodorsal nerve	C6 - C8
Elevation of the shoulder		
Trapezius	Accessory nerve	C3, 4
Levator scapulae	Dorsal scapular nerve	C3 - C5
Depression of the shoulder		
Trapezius	Accessory nerve	C3, 4
Adduction of the scapula		
Trapezius	Accessory nerve	C3, 4
Rhomboideus major	Dorsal scapular nerve	C4, 5

Manipulation of the shoulder joint

For treatment purposes the shoulder joint is manipulated in the four movements described below supplementing the action of the weaker muscles and relaxing spasticity (see Figs 3.3, 3.4, 3.5 and 3.6).

1. Elevation of the upper limb so that it is straight with the hand pointing towards the ceiling. From a position where the upper limb is beside the trunk with the hand pointing towards the floor, the normal range of movement in completing full elevation is through an arc of 180° (see Fig. 3.3).

2. Brushing the forehead with upper part of the forearm. In this the shoulder and upper arm elevate to about 130° with 90° of flexion at the elbow joint, and then abduction at the shoulder joint to 45°. The upper part of the forearm brushes across the forehead, and finally, the arm moves outward (abduction) to maximum range. For treatment repeat this 20 to 30 times in one session. For assessment purposes, if the upper part of forearm cannot touch the forehead that is a positive finding. Manipulative treatment involves percussion, pressing points, moving the shoulder joint, etc., until the finding is negative. (See Fig. 3.4.)

3. Touching the opposite ear with the fingers by stretching the arm behind the head (see Fig. 3.5). To start the movement, elevate the arm up to about 130°, externally rotate the shoulder joint, and then with the arm abducted with elbow joint flexion of 90°, put the hand and arm behind the head and neck to touch the opposite ear with the fingers.

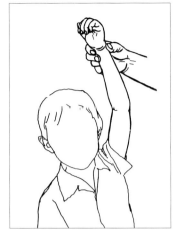

Fig. 3.3 Manipulation of the shoulder joint: raising the upper limb

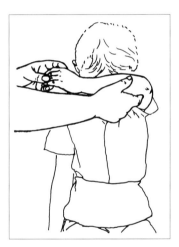

Fig. 3.4 Manipulation of the shoulder joint: brushing the forehead with the upper part of the forearm

4. Touching the spine with the thumb. The arm moves backward to maximum range, and then, flexing the elbow to 90°, with rotation of the shoulder joint, the thumb naturally touches the spine. Normally it can reach between the eighth and the fourth thoracic vertebra (see Fig. 3.6).

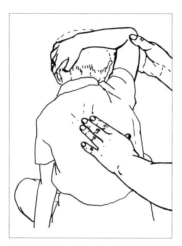

Fig. 3.5 Manipulation of the shoulder joint: touching the opposite ear with the fingers by stretching the arm behind the head

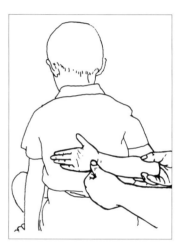

Fig. 3.6 Manipulation of the shoulder joint: touching the spine with the thumb

FOREARM SUPINATION

Limitation of forearm supination is a very common defect in patients with cerebral birth injury. It occurred in 27 (90%) of the 30 cases attending our Melbourne clinic.

The causes of disturbance of forearm supination involve spasticity of the pronator muscles of the forearm such as the Brachioradialis, Pronator teres, and Pronator quadratus. The Supinator may show spasticity at the same time. The forearm is not contracted in supination position but in pronation because the pronator group occupies a dominant position over the supinators in the forearm.

The natural or rest position of the forearm may be observed in a person who falls into a deep sleep: the arms are slightly abducted, the elbow joint may be straight or flexed, the forearm is in pronation, and the fingers are slightly flexed. These are rest positions of the human body. After injury or any pathological changes in the central nervous system, or locally in the arm, the affected limb is always kept in the natural rest position.

Inability to supinate the forearm results in the loss of hand function: the patient is unable to feed himself, touch his face, wash and dress, write, etc. If asked to hold something with the affected hand, it can be seen that he can put his arm backward but not upward or forward. This is due to spasm of the pronator.

A question often asked is why apply manipulation on the forearm supinator? In the case of cerebral palsy, spasticity may occur in both the pronators and supinators. The purpose of treatment is to relieve muscle spasm and regulate the balance of these two antagonist muscle groups.

The treatment should involve manipulation on the supinator muscle group; at the same time the upper and lower radioulnar joints should be moved.

Correction of forearm supination

• **Treatment**

1. Percussion along the anterior and posterior aspects of the forearm, to relax the increased muscle tone and to promote blood circulation in this area.
2. Pressing the forearm points 5 to 6 times on each point in one treatment:

• Jihui (Martial art point) (see Fig. 2.3).
• Sidu (SJ 9). Location: on the posterior surface of the forearm, 15 cm below the olecranon, between the radius and ulna (see Fig. 2.2).
• Ximen (P4). Location: 15 cm above the transverse flexion crease of the wrist, on the line connecting Quze (P3) and Daling (P7)), between the tendons of the Palmaris longus and Flexor carpi radialis muscles (see Fig. 2.1).
• Jianshi (P5). Location: 9 cm above the transverse flexion crease of the wrist, between the tendons of the Palmaris longus and Flexor carpi radialis muscles (see Fig. 2.1).
• Waiguan (SJ 5). Location: 6 cm above Yangchi (SJ 4), between the radius and ulna (see Fig. 2.3).

- Yangchi (SJ 4). Location: on the extension creases on the dorsum of the wrist, in the depression lateral to the tendon of the Extensor digitorum muscle (see Fig. 2.2).

3. Rotational manipulation of the forearm. Flex the elbow joint to 90°. The practitioner holds the posterior part of the patient's elbow joint with one hand, and rotates the lower part of the forearm with the other hand, turning the forearm clockwise and anticlockwise. Repeat 20 to 30 times for one treatment. (See Fig. 3.7.)

4. External fixation. This is a very useful form of treatment for severe conditions. Usually, a removable splint made of plastic or plaster is applied after 4 to 6 weeks of treatment. A removable splint allows the therapy to continue thus avoiding muscle wasting and deterioration of muscle tone. The length of the splint should be from the mid part of the arm to the tips of the fingers. The elbow joint should be flexed to 90°, the forearm rotated backward to the maximum, the thumb abducted fully and the fingers in straight position. The splint is applied on the anterior aspect of the forearm continuing beyond the posterior aspect of the elbow joint to the upper arm. The period of fixation may be short (3-4 weeks), or longer (until the deformity is corrected). Care should be taken to avoid any pressure damage from the splint.

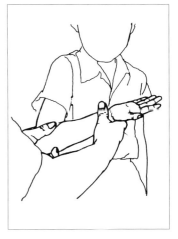

Fig. 3.7 Rotating the forearm to correct disturbance of supination

PROBLEMS OF WRIST AND HAND

There is a proverb 'Both hands are omnipotent' which means that with the two hands working in harmony it is possible to do anything. It also refers to the essential function of the hands in the human body. Hand problems are a common occurrence in patients who suffer cerebral birth injury or damage associated with other brain diseases or injuries.

Clinical manifestations

Drop wrist
This often occurs in association with deformities of the thumb or finger. The causes are spasticity or contracture of the Flexors or weakness of the Extensors of wrist and fingers.

Adduction contracture of the thumb
The causes of this condition may be weakness of any or all of the Extensor pollicis longus, Extensor pollicis brevis, Abductor pollicis longus, and Abductor pollicis brevis muscles. The condition may also result from spasm of the Flexor pollicis longus, Flexor pollicis brevis, and Adductor pollicis muscles.

Clawfingers
The normal functions of the affected fingers are limited or lost due to spasticity in the fingers resulting in difficulty or inability in grasping (see Fig. 3.11).

Thalamic   hand

With unilateral lesions of the thalamus, the contralateral hand is held in an abnormal posture. In patients with thalamic lesions, the forearm is pronated, the wrist is flexed, and the fingers are flexed at the metacarpophalangeal joints, and extended at the interphalangeal joints. The fingers can move, but the movements are limited and slow. The condition is due to altered muscle tone in the different muscle groups.

Finger movement

When the patient cannot draw the index, ring and little fingers close to the middle finger in the plane of the palm of the hand (movements described as adduction of the fingers), the condition is due to paralysis or stiffness of the Palmar interosseous muscles; when the patient cannot draw the index, ring and little fingers in the opposite direction away from the middle finger, the condition is due to paralysis or stiffness of the Dorsal interosseous muscles.

Knuckles and finger joints

Both sets of Interosseous muscles also produce flexion at the metacarpophalangeal joints and proximal and distal extension of the interphalangeal joints, movements which are lost if the muscles are paralysed.

Therapy for disturbance of wrist and hand function

• Treatment

1. Percussion along the anterior and posterior aspects of forearm, wrist and hand (palmar and dorsal aspects) to relax muscle tone and promote blood circulation.

2. Pressing the following points 5 to 6 times on each point in one treatment:

- Jihui (Martial Art point) (see Fig 2.3).
- Sidu (SJ 9). Location: on the lateral side of the forearm, 15 cm below the olecranon, between the radius and ulna (see Fig. 2.2).
- Ximen (P4). Location: 15 cm above the transverse crease of the wrist, on the line connecting Quze (P3) and Daling (P7) (Location: between the tendons of the Palmaris longus and the Flexor carpi radialis muscles) (see Fig. 2.1).
- Jianshi (P5). Location: 9 cm above the transverse crease of the wrist, between the tendons of the Palmaris longus and the Flexor carpi radialis muscles (see Fig. 2.1).
- Waiguan (SJ 5). Location: 6 cm above Yangchi (SJ 4), between the radius and ulna (see Fig.2.3).
- Yangchi (SJ 4). Location: on the transverse crease of the dorsum of the wrist, in the depression lateral to the tendon of the Extensor digitorum muscle (see Fig. 2.2).
- Yangxi (LI 5). Location: on the radial side of the wrist. When the thumb is fully extended, it is in the depression between the tendons of Extensor pollicis longus and brevis (see Fig. 2.3). Pressure at this point is used to relax flexion contracture of the thumb.

- Hegu (LI 4). Location: on the dorsum of the hand, between the first and second metacarpal bones, at approximately the mid-point of the second metacarpal bone on the radial side (see Fig. 2.3). Pressure is applied here for spasm, tremor, and pain in the upper limb, and weakness and motor impairment of the upper limb.
- Zhangjian (Martial Art points). Location: 1 cm above the metacarpophalangeal joint. There are three points located in each of the spaces separating the second and third, third and fourth, and fourth and fifth located metacarpal bones (see Fig. 2.2). These points are used for treatment of clawfingers, weakness and atrophy of the intrinsic muscles of the hand, and paralysis of median, ulnar, and radial nerves. (Acupressure therapy leads to (a) increased muscle tone of weak muscles and (b) a diminution of the high tone of spastic muscles).
- Zhiguanjie (Martial Art points). Location: around the proximal and distal interphalangeal joints of the index, middle, ring and little fingers (see Fig. 2.1). These points are used for treatment of clawfingers, drop wrist, weakness and atrophy of the muscles of hand and arm, paralysis of the arm, and spasm of the intrinsic muscles of the hand.
- Zhijiagen (Martial Art points). Location: at the nailfolds of thumb, index, middle, ring and little fingers. They are located just above the roots of the nails (see Fig. 2.2). The indications for use are the same as the Zhiguanjie points.

3. Correction of adduction contracture of the thumb (see Fig. 3.9 for children, and Fig. 3.12 for adults), is as follows:
   a. Percussion along the radial aspect of wrist and forearm.

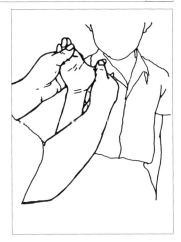

Fig. 3.8 Manipulations for correction of deformities of wrist and hand. Take the patient's hand as indicated in the figure and extend the hand, thumb, and fingers at the wrist, and metacarpophalangeal and interphalangeal joints. Massage is given on the palm to relax the spastic intrinsic muscles of the inner hand

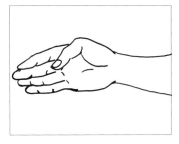

Fig. 3.9 Adduction contracture of the thumb

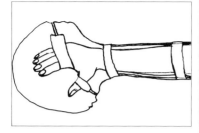

Fig. 3.10 Splint for correction of adduction contracture of the thumb, often used with children

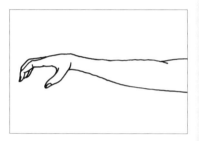

Fig. 3.11 Flexion contracture of the fingers (clawfingers)

    b. Pressing point Yangxi (LI 5) 5 to 6 times for one treatment and also point Zhijiangen (Martial Art points).

    c. Massage on the palm and thumb using thumb massage techniques (see Fig. 3.8) to relieve spasticity of inner hand muscles, including Flexor pollicis brevis, Adductor pollicis, and Opponens pollicis.

    d. Splint for correction of adduction contracture of the thumb (see Fig. 3.10). This splint is used to maintain abduction of the thumb and it may also be used for external fixation between regular functional exercise for the condition of flexion contracture of the thumb.

4. Correction of clawfingers (Fig. 3.11) is as follows:

    a. Percussion along the forearm, wrist, hand and fingers.

    b. Pressing the following points:

- Jihui (Martial Art point) (see Fig. 2.3).
- Sidu (SJ 9). Location: on the lateral side of the forearm, 15 cm below the olecranon, between the radius and ulna (see Fig. 2.2).
- Waiguan (SJ 5). Location: 6 cm above Yang chi (SJ 4), between the radius and ulna (see Fig. 2.3).
- Yangchi (SJ 4). Location: on the transverse crease of the dorsum of wrist; in the depression lateral to the tendon of Extensor digitorum (see Fig. 2.2).
- Zhiguanjie (Martial Art points). Location: on the 8 interphalangeal joints.
- Zhijiagen (Martial Art points). Location: on the 5 nailfolds over the roots of the nail.

    c. Massage using two thumbs on the palm and fingers, at the same time carrying out control led over-extension of the fingers (see Fig. 3.8).

d. Splint for correction of flexion contracture of fingers (see Fig. 3.12).

5. Functional exercises. The following functional exercises are used:

   a. Starting with the fingers apart and straight, make a fist, opening and closing the hand (see Fig. 3.13).

   b. Abduction of the thumb (see Fig. 3.14).

   c. Pushing the palms firmly together with maximal extension of wrists (see Fig. 3.15).

   d. Opposing the tip of the thumb as firmly as possible with the tips of index, middle, ring, and little fingers.

   e. Knitting, writing, picking up small objects, dressing, etc.

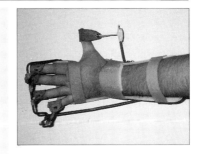

Fig. 3.12 Splint for correction of flexion contracture of the fingers, and Flexor muscles of fingers and wrist (for adults)

The practitioner prescribes exercises, their frequency, and the follow up needed to assess their results, according to the individual patient's needs.

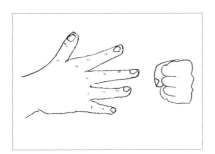

Fig. 3.13 Functional exercises for thumb and fingers. Opening and closing the hand: first opening the hand with fingers apart and straight; then making a fist

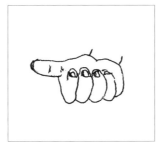

Fig. 3.14 Exercise: abduction movement of the thumb

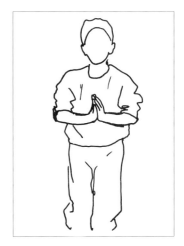

Fig. 3.15 Exercise: putting the palms together to extend the wrist

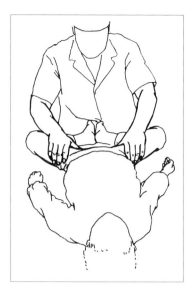

Fig. 3.16 Manipulation of the hip joint: abduction of the hip joint. For correction of adductor deformity of hip joints, the patient lies in a supine position on a bed and flexes both knee joints to 90°. The practitioner then holds the medial side of both knee joints and separates them laterally. Usually it is helpful to massage the spastic muscles on the medial aspect of the thighs

DEFORMITIES AND DYSFUNCTION OF THE LOWER LIMBS

 ## PROBLEMS OF THE HIP

Movement of the hip joint

The main muscles involved in movement of the hip joint are as follows:

Flexion - Iliopsoas, Sartorius, Rectus femoris, Tensor fasciae latae, Pectineus

Extension - Gluteus maximus, Biceps femoris, Semimembranosus, Semitendinosus

Adduction - Adductor magnus, Adductor longus, Adductor brevis, Pectineus, Gracilis

Abduction - Gluteus medius, Gluteus minimus, Gluteus maximus, Tensor fasciae latae, Sartorius

Internal rotation - Gracilis, Gluteus medius, Gluteus minimus, Tensor fasciae latae, Semitendinosus, Semimembranosus

External rotation - Iliacus, Piriformis, Obturator internus, Obturator externus, Quadratus femoris, Sartorius, Adductor magnus, Adductor longus, Adductor brevis, Biceps femoris.

Adduction contracture of the hip joint

This is due to spasticity of the hip adductors including the Adductor longus, Adductor magnus, Adductor brevis, Gracilis, and Pectineus muscles. Where the frog test is positive, the patient has major difficulty in standing, walking, and personal hygiene. Abduction of the hip joint (see Fig. 3.16), is an appropriate procedure for correction of this deformity.

Limitation of rotation of the hip joint

Limitation of internal rotation may occur due to spasm or contracture of external rotators of the hip joint such as the Iliopsoas, Obturator internus, Quadratus femoris, and the Obturator externus muscles. It is also due to weakness of internal rotators such as the Sartorius muscle. The manipulation is shown in Figure 3.17.

Limitation of external rotation may occur due to spasm or contracture of internal rotators of the hip joint. It is also due to weakness of external rotators. The manipulation is shown in Figure 3.18.

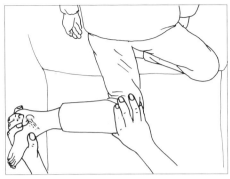

Fig. 3.17 Medial (internal) rotation of hip joint. The patient lies on a bed and flexes one hip joint and one knee joint to 90°. The practitioner holds the anterior part of the knee joint with one hand and the leg just above the ankle with the other hand, and then rotates the hip joint medially and laterally. Repeat this 20-30 times in one treatment. After this circumduction movements are carried out 20-30 times

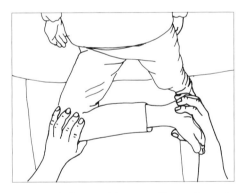

Fig. 3.18 Lateral (external) rotation of the hip joint

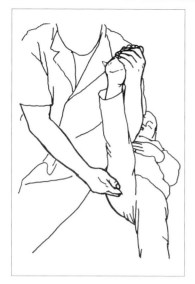

Fig. 3.19 Stretching and elevation of the lower limb and massage along the posterior aspect of the thigh with three fingers. The patient lies on the bed in a supine position. The leg is stretched and raised and placed on the practitioner's left arm. The practitioner puts his right hand on the upper portion of the patient's thigh and massages downwards towards the insertion of spastic muscles with index, middle, and ring fingers. Repeat 20-30 times.

Limitation of flexion of the hip joint

The main cause is spasticity of the Biceps femoris, Semitendinosus and Semimembranosus muscles, and in some cases it is also due to apparent weakness of flexor muscles such as the Iliopsoas, Sartorius, Rectus femoris and Tensor fasciae latae muscles. Acupressure therapy is applied as in Figure 3.19 to relax the spasm of the Hamstring muscles. Percussion and massage are applied to the weakened muscles at the anterior aspect of the thigh to increase the muscle tone of the hip flexors.

Abduction and external rotation deformity

This deformity of the hip joint often occurs due to contracture of the iliotibial tract, but in some cases it is due to weakness or paralysis of the Adductor muscles. In some patients one side is affected, but it is often found on both sides, so that when the patient lies on his back, the hip joints and legs are in the frog position.

Management involves two orthopaedic manipulations:

1. Manipulation of the iliotibial tract (see Figs 3.20 and 3.21).

2. External fixation by the use of a fish-form splint. Put the splint between the two legs and fix it with belts (see Fig. 3.58).

Contracture of Flexors of the hip joint

The clinical picture shows that the patient has difficulty walking in an upright posture. The walk is with short steps, and the hip joint partially flexes. Physically, there is difficulty with full extension at the hip joint which shows up as positive in the 4-form test. The manipulative treatment is shown in Figure 3.22.

Structural disorders of the hip joint

Several disorders of the hip joint, whether they have a developmental origin such as a congenital dislocation of the hip joint or a fracture of the neck of the femur in an elderly person following a fall, may be accompanied by relatively little or no discomfort, however some impairment of the function of the hip joint is likely to follow with signs and symptoms which provide evidence of the underlying problem. For example, in a patient with an incomplete dislocation of the hip joint the affected lower limb may be adducted with some degree of internal rotation.

It is essential that the underlying disorder is recognized and fully understood so that treatment and

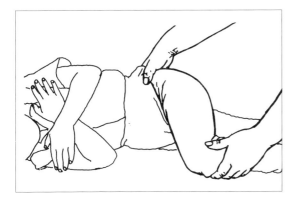

Fig. 3.20 Manipulation of the iliotibial tract. The patient lies on one side. The practitioner holds and fixes the hip bone with one hand and massages along the iliotibial tract with the other hand

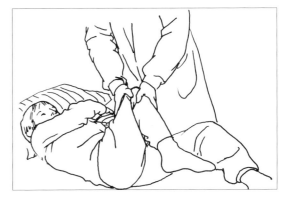

Fig. 3.21 Manipulation of the iliotibial tract: the second form

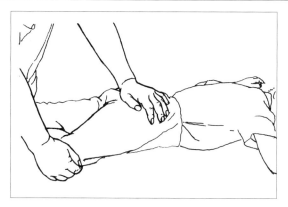

Fig. 3.22 4-form manipulation in prone position. The patient lies on the bed in a prone position. One knee joint is flexed to 90° and the limb is placed under the other in a 4-form. The practitioner presses downward on the extended leg from the gluteal region with one hand and massages along the Rectus femoris muscle with the other hand to relax the contracture of Rectus femoris and Iliopsoas muscles

rehabilitation programmes appropriate to the condition are developed and initiated at the appropriate time. These programmes will most certainly need to be directed towards maintaining effective functioning of the individual muscles and muscle groups which produce movements at the joint. Certain principles of therapy in the preceding pages for strengthening and maintaining the function of the flexor, extensor, adductor, abductor, and rotator muscles acting on the hip joint will be of benefit in restoring to a normal level the actions of those muscles whatever the nature of disorder affecting the joint. For example, the frog splint can be used for dislocation or subdislocation of the hip joint (see Figs 3.55 and 3.56), and is effective before 5 years of age.

DEFORMITIES AND CONTRACTURES OF THE KNEE JOINT

Movement of the knee joint

The muscles involved in movement of the knee joint are as follows:

Flexion - Gracilis, Politeus, Gastrocnemius, Soleus, Biceps femoris, Semimembranosus, Semitendinosus

Extension - Quadriceps femoris, Tensor fasiae latae.

Flexion contracture of the knee joint occurs in patients who suffer cerebral birth injury. It is due to spasticity and contracture of the Hamstring muscles, (Biceps femoris, Semitendinosus, and Semimembranosus). It may also be due to contracture of Gastrocnemius and Soleus muscles, as described in detail on pages 167 and 168.

The consequences of flexion contracture of the knee joint are serious. The patient cannot support his weight on his legs and cannot walk. It is very difficult, in our experience, to correct this deformity. It is no wonder, having lost their confidence, that patients frequently do not succeed in overcoming flexion contracture of the knee joint.

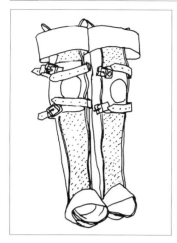

Fig. 3.23 Splints for knee and ankle joints

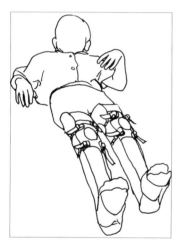

Fig. 3.24 Fixation of the knees and ankles with splints

Correction of flexion contracture of the knee

• Treatment

1. Percussion along the thigh and leg.

2. With the patient in the supine position, elevation of the lower limb with the knee joint extended as fully as possible (see Fig. 3.19).

3. Relaxation of the contracted muscles (Hamstrings and Gastrocnemius, and Soleus) by percussion and massage directly on the individual tendons and muscles, with the patient in the prone position and the knee joint in a position of maximal passive extension.

4. Flexing with a splint. This may be used for external fixation between periods of manipulation therapy. The splint should maintain the knee joint in the position of extension, with dorsal flexion of the ankle joint more than 90° (see Figs 3.23 and 3.24).

5. Manipulation of the knee joint. The patient is in the supine position. The practitioner places the patient's affected leg on his flexed forearm and then presses downward on the knee joint using both hands, and at the same time elevates the leg below the knee with the flexed arm (see Fig. 3.25). Do this 20-30 times in one treatment. After manipulation, the splint can be applied. The practitioner should be careful to avoid any pressure or damage from the splint. Some patients with less pronounced deformity may only need use the splint (see Fig. 3.26) to correct flexion contracture of the knee joint.

6. Standing exercises (see Figs 3.27, 3.28, 3.29, 3.30, 3.31, 3.32 and 3.33). Squatting exercises (see Figs 3.43, 3.44). Walking exercises (see Figs 3.34, 3.35, 3.40). Jumping exercises (see Figs 3.41, 3.42). There is a range of options in these exercises, the most suitable should be selected for specific cases.

Correction of over extension of the knee joint

This deformity often occurs in patients with sequelae of poliomyelitis, but it also occurs, although less frequently, in patients who have cerebral palsy. The treatment is also very difficult in clinical practice, and the results of the curative therapy are unsatisfactory.

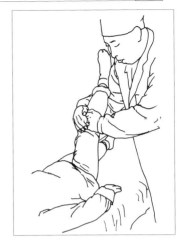

Fig. 3.25 Manipulation for correction of flexion contracture of the knee joint

- **Treatment**

1. Percussion generally on the thigh and leg, to increase the muscle tone of the Hamstring, and Gastrocnemius and Soleus muscles.

2. Pressing the following points 5 to 6 times in one treatment:

- Huantiao (G30). Location: at the junction of the lateral third and medial two-thirds of a line between the greater trochanter and the hiatus of the sacrum. When locating the point, put the patient in the lateral recumbent position with the thigh flexed (see Fig. 2.2).
- Chengfu (B36). Location: in the middle of the transverse gluteal fold. Locate the point with the patient in the prone position (see Fig. 2.2).
- Yinmen (B37). Location: 18 cm below Chengfu (B36) on the line joining Chengfu and Weizhong (B40) (see Fig. 2.2).

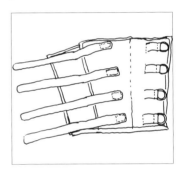

Fig. 3.26 Splint for correction of flexion contracture of the knee joint

- Weizhong (B40). Location: at the midpoint of the transverse crease of the popliteal fossa, between the tendons of the the the Biceps femoris and Semitendinous muscles (see Fig. 2.2).
- Chengshan (B57). Location: directly below the muscle belly of the Gastrocnemius on the line joining Weizhong (B40) and point Genjian (Martial Art point), about 24 cm below Weizhong (see Fig. 2.2).
- Genjian (Martial Art point). Location: at the back of the heel just on the tubercle of the calcaneus, at the insertion of the Tendo calcaneus (see Fig. 2.2).

3. The standing, squatting and walking exercises (see Figs 3.27 - 3.44).

4. Adduction, abduction, flexion, and extension manipulation of the hip joints with or without resistance.

5. Massage (grasping) of the muscle groups of the gluteal region, the thigh (4 aspects, i.e., anterior, posterior, medial and lateral), and the leg (2 aspects, i.e., antero-lateral, posterior).

6. Standing exercises (see Figs 3.27 - 3.33). Standing against a corner (see Fig. 3.27).

7. External fixation in the form of a splint for adduction contracture may also help correct over extension of the knee joint.

CASE NOTE — *Male, aged 3 years*

The patient was diagnosed as having cerebral birth injury with quadriplegia, adduction contracture of both hip joints, an eversion (valgus) deformity of the foot on both sides, an inability to sit or stand, and over-extended knee joints in both legs. The frog splint (Fig. 3.55) was applied in order to correct hip joint adduction contracture. After 3 weeks, it was found to have corrected the over-extended knee joints also.

Exercises

Figures 3.27 to 3.44 illustrate standing, squatting, and walking exercises. There is a range of options in these exercises; the most suitable should be selected for specific cases.

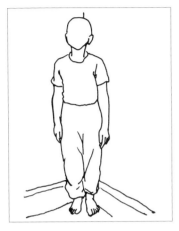

Fig. 3.27 Standing against a corner

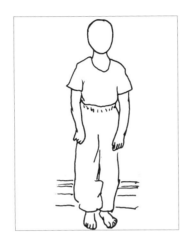

Fig. 3.28 Standing against a wall

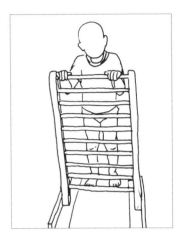

Fig. 3.29 Standing with the support of a frame: first form

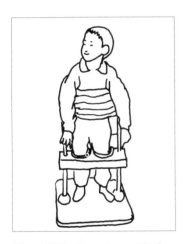

Fig. 3.30 Standing with the support of a frame: second form

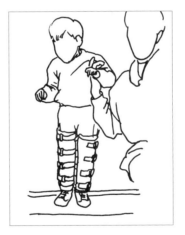

Fig. 3.31 Standing with hand support

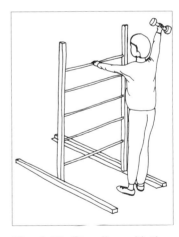

Fig. 3.32 Standing with the support of one hand on a frame

Exercises cont.

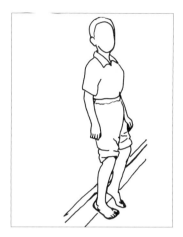

Fig. 3.33 Standing on tip toes. This exercise is to increase the muscle tone of the lower limbs

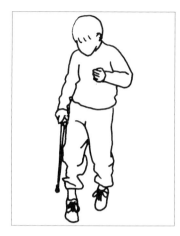

Fig. 3.34 Walking with a stick

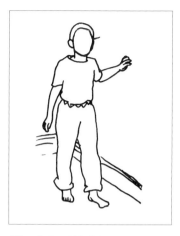

Fig. 3.35 Walking with the support of a wall

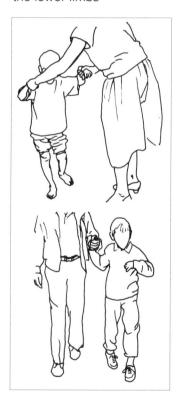

Fig. 3.36 Walking with the support of a hand

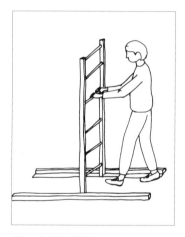

Fig. 3.37 Walking with a frame support: first form

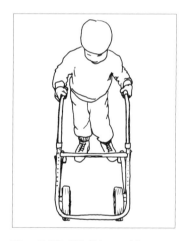

Fig. 3.38 Walking with a frame support: second form

Exercises cont.

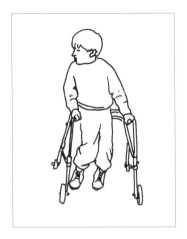

Fig. 3.39 Walking with a frame support: third form

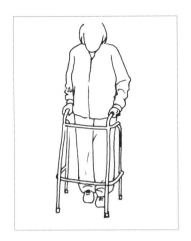

Fig. 3.40 Walking with a frame support: fourth form

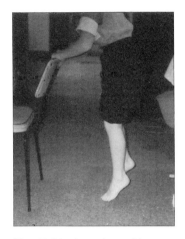

Fig. 3.41 Jumping with support

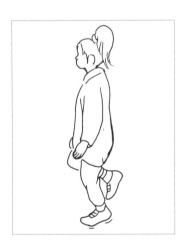

Fig. 3.42 Hopping without support

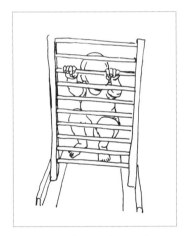

Fig. 3.43 Squatting with the support of a frame

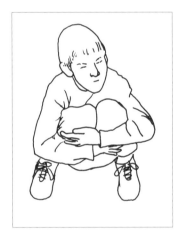

Fig. 3.44 Squatting without support

PROBLEMS OF THE ANKLE JOINT AND FOOT

Movement of the ankle joint and foot

The muscles involved in movement of the ankle joint are as follows:

Dorsiflexion - Tibialis anterior, Extensor digitorum longus, Extensor hallucis longus

Plantar flexion - Tibialis posterior, Flexor digitorum longus, Flexor hallucis longus

Inversion of the foot - Tibialis anterior, Tibialis posterior

Eversion of the foot - Peroneus longus, Peroneus brevis.

The above muscles also produce movements at either the joints of the foot or toes, or both, when they are assisted by other small intrinsic muscles of the foot.

• Normal movements

The only movements at the ankle joint are *plantar flexion* (the movement when the heel is lifted off the ground) and *dorsiflexion* (the movement associated with walking on the heel of the foot).

The foot comprises several bones and joints. Functionally the subtalar and transverse tarsal joints form a single joint for torsion or rotary movements of the foot which occur below the talus, the only bone of the foot entering into the ankle joint. The torsion movements - known as *inversion* and *eversion* - occur around an oblique axis directed forwards upwards and medially.

With inversion, the sole of the foot is rotated inwards and is said to be in a *varus* position. The movement is freer during plantar flexion at the ankle joint and is produced mainly by Tibialis anterior and Tibialis posterior muscles.

With eversion, the sole of the foot is directed downwards and slightly outwards and is said to be in a *valgus* position. The movement is freer during dorsiflexion and is produced mainly by Peroneus longus and Peroneus brevis muscles.

Clinical considerations

When the foot adopts certain abnormal positions as a result of paralysis or congenital defect, the condition is referred to as club foot or talipes. Various types of talipes are described according to the position of the foot:

1. Talipes equinus or 'drop foot' (in plantar flexion)

2. Talipes calcaneus (in dorsiflexion)

3. Talipes varus (inversion)

4. Talipes valgus (eversion)

5. Combinations of these such as talipes equinovarus when the Peroneus longus and brevis muscles are paralysed through damage to the common peroneal nerve.

Ankle joints and feet occupy an important place in the stabilization of posture and weight in the human body. A whole series of deformities occur in patients with cerebral birth injury in which the normal functions of ankle joint, feet, and even the whole body are deeply disturbed. The treatment of these deformities is important because every therapeutic gain, however minor, has great significance for the patients and their families. The specific deformities of ankle joint and foot in patients with the sequelae of cerebral birth injury are discussed next.

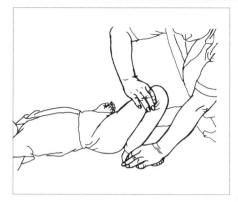

Fig. 3.45 Correction of drop foot by compression over the knee. The patient lies in a supine position on the examination table with the knee in 90° flexion. The practitioner pushes down just above the knee with one hand and pushes forcibly backward from the front of the ankle with the other hand. Repeat 20-30 times in one treatment

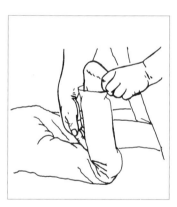

Fig. 3.46 Correction of drop foot by pressure on sole of the foot and massage over posterior aspect of the leg. The patient lies in a prone position with the knee in 90° flexion. The practitioner pushes down on the sole of the patient's foot and massages with three fingers along the back of the calf

Drop foot

In this condition the foot is in a position of plantar flexion only at the ankle joint; the foot is not inverted or everted. It may be the result of spasm of the Gastrocnemius and Soleus muscles. It may also be due to weakness of the Tibialis anterior, Extensor hallucis longus, and Extensor digitorum longus muscles.

• **Treatment**

1. Percussion along the anterolateral aspects of the leg and ankle.

2. Pressing the following points 5-6 times in one treatment:

• Jiexi (S41) (see Fig. 2.1).
• Fenglong (S40) (see Fig. 2.3).

3. Manipulations. For correction of drop foot these are by compression over the knee (see Fig. 3.45), application of pressure to the sole of the foot and massage of the posterior aspect of the leg (see Fig. 3.46). External fixation can be used (see Figs 3.23 and 3.24).

Equinovarus

Equinovarus is the deformity of the ankle and foot which combines drop foot with inversion due to contracture of the Tibialis anterior and Tibialis posterior muscles. It occurs commonly in patients with cerebral birth injury, and also in brain damage due to stroke or other brain diseases. For acupressure treatment of equinovarus please refer to page 171.

Equinovalgus

This deformity also often occurs in patients with cerebral birth injury and other brain lesions. The clinical picture shows drop foot combined with everted rotation and deformity of the ankle and tarsal joints. It is due to contracture of the Gastrocnemius and Soleus muscles or weakness of the Peroneus longus and Peroneus brevis muscles.

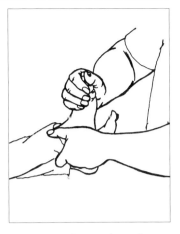

Fig. 3.47 Correction of equinovarus or equinovalgus by pulling the forefoot

• **Treatment**

1. Percussion along the lateral aspect of the leg, and massage directly on the Peroneus muscles to increase muscle tone.

2. Application of pressure to the sole of the foot and massage over posterior aspect of the calf, to relieve spasm of the Gastrocnemius and Soleus muscles (see Fig. 3.46).
   Ask the patient to lie in the prone position to carry out these manipulations.

3. Pulling on the front part of the foot to correct the everted deformity of the ankle and tarsal joints (see Fig. 3.47). External fixation can be used (see Figs 3.23 and 3.24). Pulling the forefoot is also used to correct the inverted deformity of the ankle and tarsal joints in patients with equinovarus.

Valgus deformity of the foot

This deformity is often found in patients with cerebral birth injury, and also in patients following the onset of poliomyelitis. It may be the result of spasm or contracture of the Peroneus longus and Peroneus brevis muscles, and may also be due to weakness of the Tibialis anterior and Tibialis posterior muscles, both of which invert the foot.

• **Treatment**

1. Percussion and massage along the anterolateral aspect of the leg to relieve muscle spasm.

2. Pressing the following points:

• Zusanli (S36). Location: in the Tibialis anterior muscle 9 cm below the upper border of the tibia, one finger's breadth from the anterior margin of the tibia (see Fig. 2.3).
• Yanglingquan (G34). Location: in the depression anterior and inferior to the head of the fibula (see Fig. 2.3).
• Fenglong (S40). Location: 24 cm above the external malleolus in an adult of average height (see Fig. 2.3).
• Zulinqi (G41). Location: in the depression distal to the junction of the fourth and fifth metatarsal bones, on the lateral side of the tendon of Extensor digitorum longus passing to the little toe of the foot (see Fig. 2.3). Press each point 5 to 6 times for one treatment.

3. After manipulative treatment, external fixation is applied with the foot slightly flexed at the ankle joint, using a splint applied to the back of the calf and extending from the level of the head of the fibula, around the heel, and along the sole of the foot as far as the tips of the toes. The splint can be used continuously for one to two months or more. It can be taken off for treatment, and bathing or showering.

Clawfoot

Clawfoot appears often with a combination of equinovarus or equinovalgus. Consequently manipulations similar to those mentioned above for equinovarus or equinovalgus are appropriate. In addition, compression of the arch of the foot with two hands can be used (see Fig. 3.48).

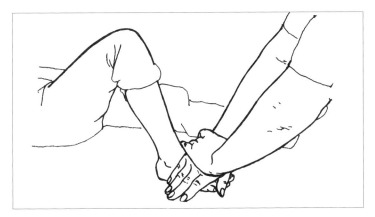

Fig. 3.48 Compression of the arch of the foot with two hands for correction of clawfoot. Perform this once only in each treatment

POSTURAL PROBLEMS

Weakness of the spinal column

This condition is often found in patients with general weakness or malnutrition, in patients who are unable to sit upright or have limited movement, and in patients whose spinal column is in a flexed position.

• Treatment

1. To correct the flexed position, the patient sits on the treatment table. The parent sits beside the patient with one hand holding down the thighs against the table and the other hand supporting the lower back. The practitioner assists movement of the patient from the sitting to the lying position. Repeat 5 to 10 times.

2. In the supine position (lying on the back) the patient arches and flattens the back. The parent places one or two hands under the patient's back to support and assist this exercise. Repeat 5 to 10 times (see Fig. 3.49).

3. The patient rolls over into the prone position. The practitioner presses along both sides of the spine (5-10 times), and presses points Yaoyan (Extra 37) (see Fig. 2.2) 4 to 5 times in sitting or prone position.

4. Bridge-form exercises (see Figs 3.49 and 3.50).

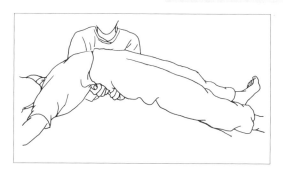

Fig. 3.49 Bridge-form exercise with support

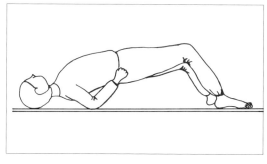

Fig. 3.50 Bridge-form exercise for the spinal column

Inability to sit up

Normally children are physically able to sit up at 20 weeks of age. Inability to sit occurs in patients with sequelae of cerebral birth injury and is caused by spasticity or contracture of the muscles around the hips. Infrequently functional disturbance of the knee joints will also affect the ability to sit.

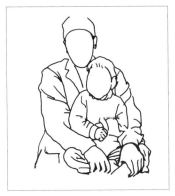

Fig. 3.51 Pressure on the back for sitting. Ask the patient to sit with crossed legs on the table. The practitioner's hands press on the patient's knees and the chest provides downward pressure on the back and forward flexion for relaxation of the spastic muscles around the hip joints

• **Treatment**

Management for inability to sit is as follows:

1. Pressure on the back for sitting (see Fig. 3.51).

2. Sitting exercises. The patient sits with the support of a frame when very weak (see Fig. 3.52).

3. Crossed leg sitting. This is an exercise of benefit to children with adduction contracture of the hip joints and limitation of external rotation of the hip joints, conditions which sometimes are associated with functional disturbance of the knee joints and valgus (see Fig. 3.53).

4. The W (M)-form sitting position is useful exercise for children with difficulty in adducting the thighs at the hip joints, and with equinovarus and iliotibial tract contracture. The patient's feet are placed in the everted position (see Fig. 3.54).

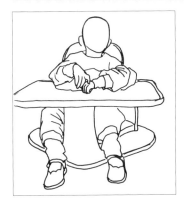

Fig. 3.52 Sitting with the support of a frame

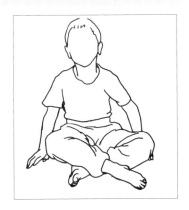

Fig. 3.53 Crossed legs sitting exercise

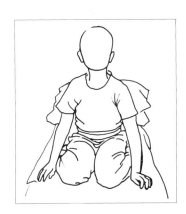

Fig. 3.54 W (M) form sitting

Inability to stand and walk

This may be due to weakness of muscles around the pelvis and in the lower limbs, or damage to the brain or cerebellum.

• Treatment

1. Pressing the following points in the gluteal region and the lower limbs:

• Huantiao (G30). Location: at the junction of the lateral third and medial two-thirds of a line between the great trochanter and the hiatus of the sacrum (see Fig. 2.2). When locating the point put the patient in lateral recumbent position with the thigh flexed.
• Chengfu (B36). Location: in the middle of the transverse gluteal fold (see Fig. 2.2). Locate the point with the patient in the prone position.
• Yinmen (B37). Location: 18 cm below Chengfu (B36), on the line joining Chengfu and Weizhong (B40) (see Fig. 2.2).
• Weizhong (B40). Location: at the midpoint of the transverse crease of the popliteal fossa, between the tendons of the Biceps femoris and Semitendinosus muscles (see Fig. 2.2).
• Chengshan (B57). Location: directly below the belly of the Gastrocnemius muscle, on the line joining Weizhong (B40) and the Tendo calcaneus (Achilles tendon) (see Fig. 2.2).
• Genjian (MA point). Location: just on the tubercle of the calcaneus, at the insertion of the Tendo calcaneus (Achilles tendon) (see Fig. 2.2).
• Biguan (S31). Location: at the crossing point of the line drawn directly down from the anterior superior iliac spine and the line level with the lower border of the symphysis pubis, in the depression on the lateral side of the Sartorius muscle when the thigh is flexed (see Fig. 2.1).

- Jimen (SP 11). Location: 18 cm above Xiehai (SP 10) on the line drawn from Xuehai (SP 10) to Chongmen (SP 12) (see Fig. 2.3).
- Futu (S32). Location: In the Rectus femoris muscle on a line connecting the anterior superior iliac spine and the lateral border of the patella, 18 cm above the laterosuperior border of the patella (see Fig. 2.1).
- Zusanli (S36). Location: In the Tibialis anterior muscle 9 cm below Dubi (S35) one finger-breadth from the anterior border of the tibia (see Fig. 2.3).
- Fenglong (S40). Location: In an adult of average height 24 cm superior to the lateral malleolus about one finger breadth lateral to Tiaokou (S38) (see Fig. 2.3).
- Lougu (SP 7). Location: 9cm above Sanyinjiao (SP 6), on the line joining the tip of the medial malleolus and Yinlingquan (SP 9) (see Fig. 2.3).

2. Adduction, abduction, flexion and extension movements of hip joints with or without resistance. Grasp and gently knead the muscle groups of the gluteal region, thigh (on its four aspects - anterior, posterior, medial and lateral), and leg (on its two aspects - antero-lateral, posterior).

Correction of scissor legs

Many factors may cause the deformity of scissor legs but the principal one is adduction contracture of the Adductor muscles of the thigh. For children, clinically we often manipulate the thighs so that they are abducted to the full range of normal movement and then use the frog splint (see Figs 3.55 and 3.56) as an external fixation for a few hours during the day or at night time (see Fig. 3.16). External rotation may also be used (see Fig. 3.57).

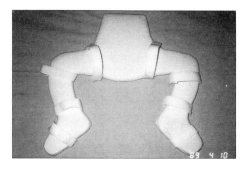

Fig. 3.55 Frog splint

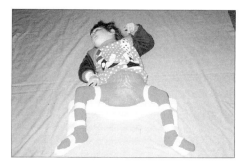

Fig. 3.56 Patient with frog splint

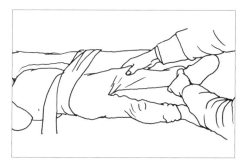

Fig. 3.57 External rotation of the lower limb for correction of scissor legs

Fish form splint

Some patients with cerebral birth injury have other deformities of the legs which may be corrected at the same time. We often use the fish form splint (see Fig. 3.58).

Indications for use of fish form splint are as follows:

- O-form deformity of legs
- X-form deformity of legs
- Abduction deformity of hip joints.
- Eversion deformity of knee joints
- Inversion deformity of knee joints.
  The fish form splint is useful in children under 5 years of age.
  Points for attention in practice are as follows:
- The belt should not be too tight.
- Apply the splint intermittently. It is used at night and during daytime rest.
- Avoid compression of the common peroneal nerve, which passes around the neck of the fibula to the outer muscles on the anterior and lateral aspects of the leg.
- The splint should be used until the deformities are corrected.

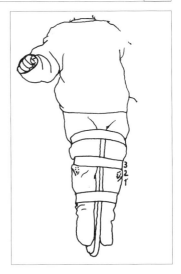

Fig. 3.58 Fish-form splint: 1. common peroneal nerve; 2. head of the fibula; 3. belt of the splint

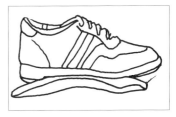

Fig. 3.59 Pad for correction of flat foot and valgus

Orthotic footwear

Consultation with a podiatrist may be required regarding provision of padded footwear to assist with correction of flat foot and valgus (see Fig. 3.59).

VISUAL DEFICITS

Pathological changes may occur in any part of the optic and visual reflex pathways in patients with cerebral birth injury. Localization of a lesion may involve the visual cortex (primary and/or secondary visual areas); midbrain; pons and medulla oblongata. Lesions of the primary visual area, in the posterior part of one calcarine sulcus result in a loss of sight in the opposite visual field, i.e., crossed homonymous hemianopia. The following clinical defects should be understood.

Lesions of the upper half of one primary visual area, i.e., the area above the calcarine sulcus, result in inferior quadrantic hemianopia, whereas lesions involving one visual area below the calcarine sulcus result in superior quadrantic hemianopia. Lesions of the occipital pole produce central scotomas. Lesions of the secondary visual area (around the primary visual area) result in a loss of ability to recognize objects seen in the opposite field of vision. The reason for this is that the area of cortex that stores past visual experiences has been lost. Lesions involving the optic nerve result in total blindness of the homolateral side; lesions involving the left optic tract result in left sided honomymous hemianopia; lesions involving the optic chiasma result in bitemporal heteronymous hemianopia and lesions involving the lateral half of the optic chiasma result in nasal hemianopia.

In addition, there are three pairs of cranial nerves which need to be understood in relation to movement of the eyeball: the oculomotor nerve (III cranial nerve) originates from the midbrain, the superior ramus supplies Superior rectus and Levator palpebrae superioris muscles; the inferior ramus supplies the Inferior and Medial rectus muscles and the Inferior oblique muscle. The trochlear nerve (IV cranial nerve) originates from the midbrain and

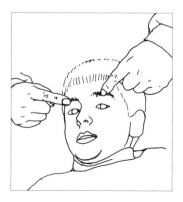

Fig. 3.60 Pressing point Jingming (B1)

Fig. 3.61 Pressing point Yuyao (Extra 3)

supplies the Superior oblique muscle. The abducent nerve (VI cranial nerve) originates from the upper portion of the medulla oblongata below the pons and supplies the Lateral rectus muscle of the eyeball. Lesions involving any one of these three nerves result in disturbance of eyeball movement.

Involvement of visual function in patients with cerebral injury was found in 12 out of 17 patients in Melbourne, which represents 70% of the cases treated. In contrast, our Institute in Beijing had about 10% incidence of visual impairment in the 150 patients with cerebral birth injury. It seems that the morbidity in Australian patients was much higher than in Chinese patients. The reason for the difference between the two groups is not clear; and perhaps the limited number of patients does not give a true indication. Another factor may be the make-up of the first Australian group, as there was a concentration of severe cases.

Visual deficits may also occur in cases of brain injury and cerebrovascular accident.

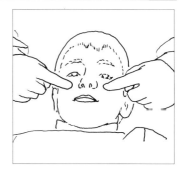

Fig. 3.62 Pressing point Chengqi (S1)

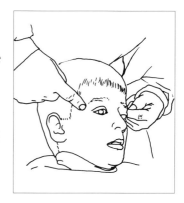

Fig. 3.63 Pressing point Sizhukong (SJ 23)

• Treatment

Treatment consists of pressing the following points 4 to 5 times every treatment:

- Jingming (B1). Location: 3 mm superior to the inner canthus (see Figs 2.1 and 3.60).
- Yuyao (Extra 3). Location: at the midpoint of the eyebrow (see Figs 2.1 and 3.61).
- Chengqi (S1). Location: with the eyes looking straight forward, the point is directly below the pupil, between the eyeball and the infraorbital ridge (see Figs 2.1 and 3.62).
- Sizhukong (SJ 23). Location: in the depression at the lateral end of the eyebrow (see Figs 2.1 and 3.63).
- Fengchi (G20). Location: in the depression between the upper portion of the Sternomastoid and Trapezius muscles, on the same level as Fengfu (see Figs 2.2 and 3.64).

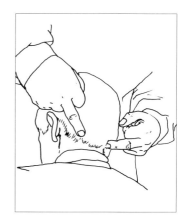

Fig. 3.64 Pressing point Fenchi (G20)

The technique of acupressure therapy was used with one session daily, or every other day, for 8 to 12 weeks in one course.

The points for attention in practice are that the patient should lie quietly in a supine position and the head should be held securely to avoid eye injury.

Case studies are presented in Table 3.2.

Table 3.2 Results of treatment of cerebral birth injury patients with visual problems

Sex	Age (yrs) (mths)	Problem	Sessions	Results
M	5y 6m	Strabismus both sides	66	Improved
M	4y 6m	Optic atrophy, strong autistic avoidance pattern	70	Patient using vision more of his own accord. Responds to light and sound, follows objects, eye contact improved. Uses vision for mobility, tracking, judging size, distance, and location of objects
F	3y 6m	Cortical blindness, both sides. Vacant glassy stare of no recognition	62	Patient's vision shows a lot of improvement, responds to light and sound. Looks at father when he speaks to her
M	3	Ventricles dilated (head ultrasound) and aqueductual stenosis (head scan). Vision weakness both sides	67	Visual function greatly improved
M	6	Intraventricular haemorrhage led to an occular squint in both eyes	70	Squint improved. Good vision
F	4y 6m	Vacant glassy stare of no recognition	70	A lot of eye contact. Looks directly at speaker, responds to sound and light and follows objects
F	2y 6m	Cortical impairment right eye	65	Improved
F	2y 6m	Optic atrophy, both eyes. Eyes roll upward, not interested in looking at toys, did not follow a light. Pale optic discs	83	Responds well to light, sound, colour, can follow objects
F	9y 6m	Vision in left eye weak. Could see a finger at a distance of 1 m	67	Sees fingers at a distance of 2 m. Vision much improved
F	2y 6m	Blind, only responded to strong light	60	Much improved, can follow some objects, responds to sound, shows interest in toys
M	4y 6m	Long-sighted, both eyes, inward turn in left eye	64	A little improved
F	5y 6m	Bilateral ventricular haemorrhage. Extensive haemorrhage into the cortical regions	84	Improved, responds to light and sound, but cannot follow objects

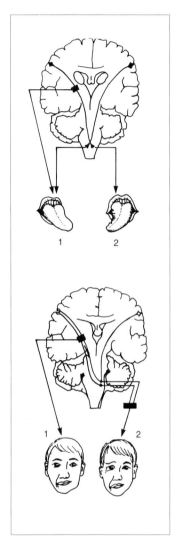

Fig. 3.65 Facial expression, defects associated with lesions of: 1. upper motor corticonuclear neurons; 2. lower motor neurons of the facial nerve

FACIAL PARALYSIS

Facial paralysis is due to injury of the facial nerve, which supplies the muscles of expression, supplies the anterior two-thirds of the tongue with taste fibres, and is secretomotor to the lacrimal, submandibular, and sublingual glands. Lesions of the facial nerve may be located within the pons of the brain, in the subarachnoid space or as it enters the temporal lobe. The part of the facial nerve nucleus that controls the muscles of the upper part of the face receives corticonuclear fibres from both cerebral hemispheres, therefore it follows that, with a lesion involving the upper motor neurons only, the muscles of the lower part of the face will be paralysed; with a lower motor neuron lesion (lesion of facial nerve motor nucleus or the facial nerve itself), all the muscles on the affected side of the face will be paralysed (see Fig. 3.65).

Clinical manifestations

The lower eyelid droops, the corner of the mouth sags, tears flow over the lower eyelid, and saliva dribbles from the corner of the mouth. The patient will be unable to close the eye or expose the teeth fully on the affected side.

• **Treatment**

1. Pressing the following points 5 to 6 times in one treatment:

- Chengqi (S1). Location: with the eyes looking straight forward, the point is directly below the pupil, between the eyeball and the infraorbital ridge (see Fig. 2.1).
- Yifeng (SJ 17). Location: posterior to the lobe of the ear, in the depression between the mandible and mastoid process (see Fig. 2.2).
- Sibai (S2). Location: below point Chengqi (S1), in the depression at the infraorbital foramen (see Fig. 2.1).
- Chuigen (MA point). Location: just below the lobe of the ear (see Figs 2.3 and 3.66).

  This treatment takes place once daily. A course of treatment comprises 40 manipulations, followed by a break of 3-4 weeks. If necessary, a second course of treatment can be given.

2. Massage along both cheeks.

3. Ask the patient to do exercises blowing out hard 20 times every hour.

4. Ask the patient to do exercises clenching the jaw 20 times every hour.

DIFFICULTY WITH SWALLOWING AND APHAGIA

Aphagia is often found in newborn babies during the first days of life. Some cases have difficulty swallowing for a long time after birth. One parent said: 'My daughter was very tight and could do nothing at all. It would take up to an hour or more just to feed her one meal.' In some children with cerebral birth injury, inhalation of saliva leads to bronchitis or aspiration pneumonia, which of course require appropriate medical treatment.

• **Treatment**

1. Suction drainage using an aspirating tube to clear the patient's throat and bronchi.

2. Massage along both sides of laryngeal region, for two purposes: the first is to relax the spasm of the small muscles; and the second is to stimulate the patient to cough up mucus and secretions from the bronchi (see Fig. 3.74).

3. Direct stimulation of the pharyngeal region with a tongue depressor, causing the patient to cough up the mucus and secretions from the bronchi, and at the same time, stimulating swallowing. All the above described methods have two actions: (a) clearing out mucus and secretions; and (b) stimulating the swallow reflex.

4. Anti-infection management involving the use of antibiotics or Chinese herbs. Sometimes we combined the two, sometimes we used only herbs.

• Herbal prescription

The following prescription of Chinese herbs might be given, for example, to a 5 year-old-child.

Flos chrysanthemi indici	野菊花	6 g
Herba taraxaci	蒲公英	10 g
Fructus forsythiae	連翹	5 g
Rhizoma pinelliae	半夏	3 g
Radix glehniae	北沙參	5 g
Radix glycyrrhizae	甘草	3 g
Radix ophiopogonis	麥冬	5 g

Mix and pour the ingredients into a small pot, then add cold water until the water covers the herbs by 3 cm. Boil for 25 minutes. Remove about 30 ml of the extract, add enough cold water to cover the herbs and boil again as above for 25 minutes more. Then take out 30 ml of the extract and mix it with the first 30 ml of the extract.

• Dosage

15 ml four times daily half an hour after meals. Continue until the infection is controlled. Store unused extract in the freezer.

CASE NOTE — *Female, aged 3 years 6 months*

This little girl had suffered cerebral birth injury, and had difficulty swallowing. She was fed with liquid and semi-liquid food for 3 years. After about 20 sessions of manipulation as mentioned above, her swallowing function was much improved.

CASE NOTE — *Male, aged 6 years*

This boy had suffered cerebral injury. He had poor control of swallowing. He inhaled saliva into his bronchi and because he could not expectorate, this led to bronchitis. The patient received acupressure therapy about 20 times, as well as administration of Chinese herbs (decoction), see above prescription (10 packs). The bronchitis was controlled. The patient was able to cough out the sputum and mucus from the bronchi and laryngeal region. His ability to swallow was greatly improved.

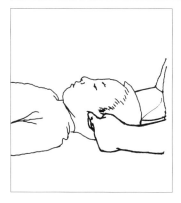

Fig. 3.66 Drooling point: pressing points Chuigen (MA point) bilaterally

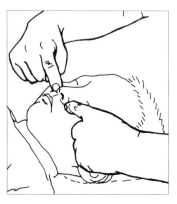

Fig. 3.67 Drooling point: pressing points Yingxiang (LI 20) both sides

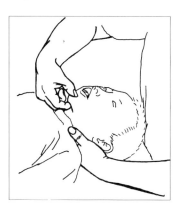

Fig. 3.68 Drooling point: pressing point Chengjiang (Ren 24) using the thumb, and pressing point Lianquan (Ren 23) using the index finger

DROOLING

Drooling often occurs in infants (it is a normal process in infants up to the age of about 15 months, and it is often seen). It also occurs in some children who suffer cerebral birth injury, in patients with previous brain injury, and in some patients following a cerebrovascular accident. It is a great problem for patients, especially as regards personal hygiene. Drooling may occur due to spasm or contracture of the muscles controlling movements of the lips, the tongue, and the lower jaw. Drooling may also be caused by the stimulation of, or some injury to, the nerves controlling secretion from the salivary glands, discussed below.

Parotid gland
Parasympathetic secretomotor fibres from the inferior salivary nucleus of the glossopharyngeal nerve supply the gland. The preganglionic nerve fibres pass to the otic ganglion through the tympanic branch of the glossopharyngeal and the lesser petrosal nerve. Postganglionic fibres reach the gland through the auriculotemporal nerve. Sympathetic postganglionic fibres arise from the superior cervical sympathetic ganglion and reach the gland as a plexus of nerves around the external carotid artery.

Submandibular and sublingual glands
Parasympathetic secretomotor supply originates in the superior salilvatory nucleus of the facial nerve. The preganglionic fibres pass to the submandibular gland either directly or along the duct. Postganglionic fibres to the sublingual gland travel through the lingual nerve. Sympathetic postganglionic fibres arise from the superior cervical sympathetic ganglion and reach the glands as a

plexus of nerves around the external carotid, facial, and lingual arteries. They function as vasoconstrictor fibres.

Difficulty in swallowing may be involved, as mentioned above.

• **Treatment**

1. Pressing the following points:

• Chuigen (MA point), Location: just below the earlobe (see Figs 2.3 and 3.66).
• Yinxiang (LI 20). Location: In the nasolabial groove, at the level of the nostrils (see Figs 2.1 and 3.67).
• Chengjiang (Ren 24). Location: in the depression in the centre of the mentolabial groove (see Figs 2.1 and 3.68).
• Lianquan (Ren 23). Location: above the prominence of the larynx, in the depression above the upper border of the hyoid bone (see Figs 2.1 and 3.68).
• Jiachengjiang (Extra 8). Location: 1 unit lateral to Chengjiang (Ren 24) directly below Dicang (S4), under which can be felt the mental foremen of the mandible (see Figs 2.1 and 3.69).

2. Pinching point Dicang (S4). Location: lateral to the corner of the mouth, directly below Sibai (S2) (see Figs 2.1 and 3.70).

3. Massage on the submandibular region (see Fig. 3.71).

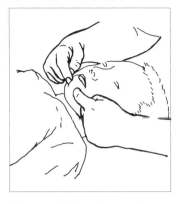

Fig. 3.69 Pressing point Jiachengjiang (Extra 8) both sides

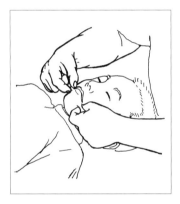

Fig. 3.70 Drooling point: pinching points Dicang (S4) both sides

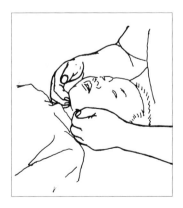

Fig. 3.71 Massage for drooling: massage on submandibular muscles

SPEECH PROBLEMS

Normal development of communication in children is as follows:

- 3-4 months, the baby sounds vary and babbling begins.
- 4-6 months, there is babbling and some intonation.
- 6-8 months, syllables begin.
- 8-12 months, double syllables are made.
- 12-20 months, the baby can speak 2-3 word phrases.
- 3 years, the infant can speak simple sentences, and asks many questions.

Unlike cases of cerebral birth injury, most brain injury and cerebrovascular accident patients will have developed and lost normal speech.

Causes of speech problems

Speech problems are the most common dysfunction in patients who suffer cerebral injury as children, or brain trauma, cerebrovascular accident, and other diseases of the brain. For an analysis of the causes of speech disturbances in patients with cerebral birth injury, the description in the following paragraphs is offered.

• Speech disturbance due to brain lesions
Destructive lesions of the motor speech area result in the loss of ability to produce speech. The motor speech area is located in the inferior frontal gyrus between the anterior and ascending rami and the ascending and posterior rami of the lateral fissure. In the majority of individuals, this area is important on the left or dominant hemisphere and damage here will result in paralysis of speech. In

those individuals where the right hemisphere is dominant, the speech area is also on the right side.

• **Speech muscle spasticity**

With speech muscle spasticity caused by lesions of the motor cortex, the severity of the clinical manifestations is different according to the condition of the brain injury. A discrete lesion of the primary motor cortex results in little change in the speech muscle tone. However, large lesions involving the primary and secondary motor areas, which are the most common, result in muscle spasm. The explanation for this is that the motor cortex gives rise to corticospinal tracts or pathways (controlling spinal motor nerves) and corticonuclear pathways (controlling cranial motor nerves) and, in addition, gives rise to extrapyramidal tracts that pass to the basal ganglia.

The corticospinal and corticonuclear pathways tend to increase muscle tone, but the extrapyramidal fibres transmit inhibitory impulses that lower muscle tone. If spasticity is present, it may be due to an inbalance between these two actions. Destruction of the secondary motor area from which the extrapyramidal pathways arise, removes the inhibitory influence and, consequently, the muscles are spastic.

• **Speech problems caused by loss of hearing**

This may be due to the lesions of the primary auditory area and also diseases of the ears.
It is extremely important to understand that delay is 'normal' for a cerebral palsied child, who cannot yet understand the meaning of sound, words and conversation, as he or she cannot see what they mean, cannot see gestures, and cannot link various stimuli from the external world.

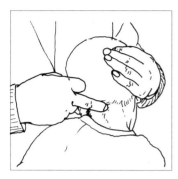

Fig. 3.72 Pressing point Yamen (DU 15)

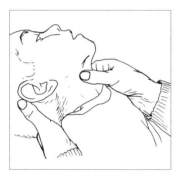

Fig. 3.73 Massage along the hyoid bone

Management of speech problems

The treatment of speech problems includes pressing points; massage along the face, mouth, and submandibular region, and massage on both sides of the laryngeal region.

• **Treatment**

1. Pressing the following points:

• Chuigen (Martial Art point) (see Fig. 3.66).
• Chengjiang (Ren 24) (see Fig. 3.68).
• Lianquan (Ren 23) (see Fig. 3.68).
• Jiachengjiang (Extra 8) (see Fig. 3.69).
• Dicang (S4) (see Fig. 3.70).
• Yamen (DU 15) (see Fig. 3.72).

2. Massage on the hyoid bone 20 times for one treatment (see Fig. 3.73).

In the submandibular region and attached to the hyoid bone, which forms a platform from which muscles of the tongue can act in producing speech, are the Digastric, Mylohyoid, Hyoglossus, Sternohyoid, Omohyoid, Stylohyoid, and Geniohyoid muscles.

3. The points for attention in clinical practice are as follows:

• Ask patient to lie on his back (in the supine position) and stay relaxed and quiet.
• Press both sides simultaneously if the point is bilateral.
• Massage the tongue muscles in the submandibular region using the index, middle and ring fingers.
• Massage the hyoid bone between the thumb and index finger.
• Administer the treatment once daily.

4. Massage on the face around the lips, and in the submandibular region. The patient sits on a stool or lies down on the examination table. The doctor stands behind the patient and massages along both cheeks using index and middle fingers with backward movements. Massage around the lips in the same way, is also part of the therapy, as is massage along the submandibular region (see Fig. 3.71). Each procedure is repeated 20 times during one treatment.

• Relief of spasm of the muscles

1. Massage along both sides of laryngeal region (see Fig. 3.74).

2. Massage on the hyoid bone (see Fig. 3.73).

• Speech exercises

Speech exercises are described on page 139.

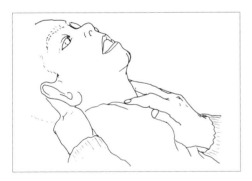

Fig. 3.74 Massage along both sides of laryngeal region

OPISTHOTONUS

This is a clinical symptom of muscle contraction due to lesions of the central nervous system. The condition exists when the muscle tone, particularly that of the muscles of the back, is greatly increased. It occurs when lesions exist that involve supraspinal centres or their descending tracts but not the corticospinal tract. It may also occur at a local spinal segmental level and may be produced by local excitation of the stretch reflex by sensory irritation, for example, spasm of back muscles secondary to a prolapsed intervertebral disc. The muscle contraction occurs suddenly, involving rigidity of the voluntary muscles situated in the limbs and on both sides of the spinal column. When the contraction begins, the four limbs are stiffened in an outstretched position and the spinal column arched due to contraction of the back muscles. The whole position is one of tension and for that reason the condition is referred to as 'opisthotonus'. The occurrence of cerebral birth injury complicated with opisthotonus is rare. The muscles involved in extension of the head, neck and spinal column connected with opisthotonus are as follows:

Splenius capitus	Longissimus cervicis
Splenius cervicis	Spinalis
Semispinalis capitis	Longissimus thoracis
Semispinalis Cervicis	Iliocostalis cervicis
Longus capitis	Iliocostalis thoracis
Longus colli	Iliocostalis lumborum
Longissimus capitis	

• **Treatment**

1. Press the point Dazhui (DU 14) and massage the soft tissue on both sides of it (see Fig. 2.2).

2. Flex the neck.

3. Massage along the posterior aspect of the root of the neck, on the Longissimus cervicis, Scalenus posterior, Longissimus capitis, Semispinalis capitis, and Semispinalis cervicis muscles.

4. Advise the patient to keep as quiet as possible and generally avoid stimulation.

5. Advise the patient that deep breathing will relieve spasms.

URINARY INCONTINENCE

Numerous factors can cause urinary incontinence or poor urinary control:

- Sequelae of cerebral birth injury, brain trauma, cerebrovascular accident and other diseases of the central nervous system
- Injuries or pathological changes of the spinal cord
- Spina bifida, encephalomyelocele
- Dysfunction of the urinary bladder wall muscle or sphincter
- Inflammation of the prepuce, urethritis, enterobiasis
- Internal tension, general weakness, old age.

Clinical manifestations

The conditions described above are due to three main causes: pathological changes in the central nervous system; local pathological changes; and influences of a psychological nature. The clinical pictures differ accordingly. Pathological changes of the central nervous system may cause the patient to present with different clinical symptoms such as the atonic, automatic reflex, and autonomous bladder.

The atonic bladder occurs during the phase of spinal shock following injury and may last from a few days to several weeks. The bladder wall muscle is relaxed, the sphincter vesicae tightly contracted, and the sphincter urethrae relaxed. The bladder becomes greatly distended and finally overflows. The automatic reflex bladder condition occurs after the patient has recovered from spinal shock, the bladder fills and empties reflexly. The sphincter vesicae and the urethral sphincter both relax. This simple reflex occurs every 1 to 4 hours. The autonomous bladder is the condition that occurs if the sacral segment of the spinal cord is destroyed. The bladder wall is flaccid, and the capacity of the bladder is greatly increased. The other symptoms are frequency of urination, urgency of micturition and incontinence of urine, or retention of urine.

Local pathological changes result in the occurrence of frequency of urination, urgency of micturition, and painful urination. These are due to stimulation caused by inflammation.

Psychological conditions: the patient with this type of bed-wetting problem usually sleeps soundly at night and has no frequency of urination, urgency or awareness of urination.

Management of urinary problems

An indwelling catheter during the early stage of injury is usually only for emergency cases, but for children with cerebral palsy the use of nappies or diapers is adequate. Acupressure manipulations for injured patients with a catheter can usually begin straight after injury. The presence of the catheter does not affect the treatment.

The points for incontinence are the same for a boy or a girl.

• **Treatment of urinary incontinence**

Routine treatment applies. The manipulations are as follows:

1. Pressing the following points with the patient in a relaxed supine position:

• Qugu (Ren 2). Location: on the midpoint of the upper border of the symphysis pubis (see Figs 2.1 and 3.75).

• Huiyin (Ren 1). Location: between the anus and the root of the scrotum in males and between anus and the posterior labial commissure in females (see Fig. 2.1).

• Qichong (S30). Location: 15cm below the umbilicus, 6 cm lateral to Qugu (Ren 2). (See Figs 2.1 and 3.76).

2. Clapping on the lower abdomen with the curved palm for 50 times for one treatment. on the points Zhongji (Ren 3) Guanyuan (Ren 4), and Qihai (Ren 6) (see Fig. 3.77).

3. Pressing the following points with the patient in a prone position:

• Yaoyan (Extra 37). Location: on both sides 4.5 cm lateral to lower border of the spinous process of the fourth lumbar vertebra (see Figs 2.2 and 3.78).

• Guanyuanshu (B26). Location: 4.5 cm lateral to the Du meridian, at the level of the lower border of the spinous process of the fifth lumar vertebra (see Fig. 2.2).

• Pangguangshe (B28). Location: 4.5 cm lateral to the Du meridian, at the level of the second posterior sacral foramen (see Figs 2.2 and 3.79).

4. After pressing the points, percussion can be given along the lower back and both gluteal regions for 5 minutes.

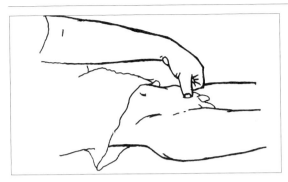

Fig. 3.75 Technique for treatment of bed wetting: pressing point Qugu (Ren 2)

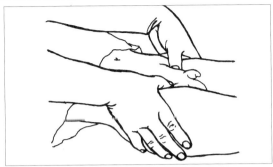

Fig. 3.76 Bed wetting point: pressing point Qichong (S30) both sides

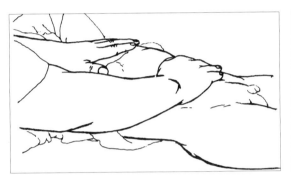

Fig. 3.77 Bed wetting point: Clapping the hand over the lower abdomen. Perform this 50 times in one treatment

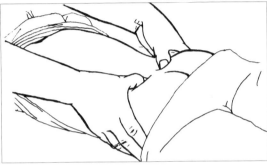

Fig. 3.78 Bed wetting point: Pressing point Yaoyan (Extra 37) both sides, 5 times in one treatment

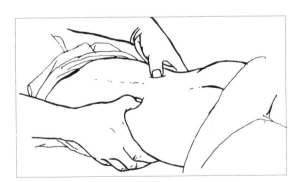

Fig. 3.79 Bed wetting point: pressing point Panguangshu (B28) both sides 5 times in one treatment

EPILEPSY

Epilepsy is a symptom in which there is a sudden transitory disturbance of the normal function of the brain. The condition is usually associated with a disturbance of normal electrical activity and in its most typical form is accompanied by seizures. Clinically, the patient does not lose consciousness in partial seizures as, in this case, the abnormality occurs in only one part of the brain. We have often found patients of cerebral birth injury had complications in this form.

In patients with generalized seizures, the abnormal activity involves large areas of the brain on both sides and the individual loses consciousness. In the majority of cases with generalized seizures, there is a sudden loss of consciousness and other symptoms such as tonic spasm, clonic contractions of the muscles and loss of control of bowel and bladder. The convulsions last from a few seconds to a few minutes.

The causes of epilepsy include scarring of the cerebral cortex following trauma such as pre- or perinatal anoxia, and cerebral tumours; however, the cause is unknown in the majority of patients with epilepsy.

• **Treatment**

1. Pressing the following points:

- Naokong (G19) (see Fig. 2.3).
- Fengchi (G20) (see Fig. 2.3).
- Daling (P7). Location: In the middle of the transverse crease of the wrist, between the tendons of the Palmaris longus and Flexor carpiradialis muscles (see Fig. 2.1).
- Neignan (P6). Location: 6 cm above thetransverse crease of the wrist, between thetendons of the Palmaris longus and the Flexor carpi radialis muscles (see Fig. 2.1).
- Dazhui (DU 14). Location: Below the spinous process of the seventh cervical vertebra, approximately at the level of the shoulders (see Fig. 2.2).
- Jiexi (S41). Location: On the dorsum of the foot, at the midpoint of the transverse crease of the ankle joint, in the depression between the tendons of the Extensor digitorum longus and Hallucis muscles, approximately at the level of the tip of the lateral malleolus (see Fig 2.1).

2. Oral administration of antiepileptic drugs - according to doctor's orders.

3. The patient should have enough rest, avoid constipation and refrain from any strong stimulation.

CHAPTER 4

CEREBRAL BIRTH INJURY

The term 'cerebral birth injury' commonly refers to a group of conditions characterised by brain and motor dysfunction resulting from: (1) antenatal injury, including brain damage of the fetus; or (2) injury during delivery; or (3) during the early post-natal period.

CAUSES

The causes of cerebral birth injury are usually external to the brain rather than inherent. Table 4.1 shows the causes in 150 cases treated at the Institute of Orthopaedics and Traumatology, Beijing.

Table 4.1 Causes of cerebral birth injury in 150 patients

Delayed birth with anoxia	62
Instrument trauma and anoxia	39
Improper manipulation	16
Surgical operation and anoxia	11
Umbilical cord round neck	10
Breech presentation	8
Abruptio placentae	4
	150

Factors during pregnancy

Among our case histories there were some children who received cerebral injuries in utero, as a result of lack of oxygen experienced by the mother and hence the fetus during pregnancy. Prematurity may also be associated with brain injury. This combination occurred in about 30% of our patients in Australia. Cerebral damage resulting in cerebral palsy has also been attributed to over-exposure to X-rays during pregnancy, and even to small amounts of radiation during the early stages of pregnancy.

Factors during delivery

Sometimes children with cerebral injury were born after a rapid labour, averaging less than 2 hours. On the other hand, some children with cerebral injury were born after a protracted labour, averaging more than 24 hours. Of the 150 brain damaged children treated in Beijing there were 11 cases who had had a difficult delivery, ending in a caesarean section, and accompanied by postnatal anoxia. There were 62 children who had suffered injury as a result of a protracted labour and anoxia.

Obstetrical difficulties resulting in brain injury, included breech presentation (a factor in 8 cases) and of prematurely separated placenta, resulting in the loss of blood and subsequent lack of oxygen (4 cases). Some parents reported to us in the clinic that during delivery the umbilical cord was found to be wound tightly around the baby's neck, sometimes once round, sometimes twice. Tragically, this problem led to a lack of blood supply to the brain, with subsequent brain injury. We had 10 cases among the 150 patients with cerebral birth injury which may have been attributable to this factor.

For a long time I had had the impression that many of the complications during childbirth which resulted in brain injuries in children were due to the obstetrical practices and techniques which had been employed. I have come to believe, however, that such an association is relatively rare. In our retrospective analysis of the 150 cases there were only 16 patients with cerebral birth injury in whom the obstetrical manipulations required during the delivery may have been a factor associated with the subsequent damage.

For example, there were 30 cases out of the 150, where cerebral birth injury followed a delayed delivery which required the use of obstetrical forceps. It was difficult clinically to distinguish between brain injury from instruments and injury due to lack of oxygen alone. It may be that both factors operated concurrently.

Delayed symptoms

It is often found in clinical practice that it is difficult to determine when damage occurs in patients who develop symptoms such as neurological deficit, collapse, apneoic episodes, convulsions and paralysis. In our experience, the clinical symptoms are delayed in these cases. The cause may be injury during pregnancy, or during delivery. The injuries may not be severe and there may be no clinical symptoms at the time. Pathological changes develop later, and it may take a few days, weeks, months, or even years for the clinical symptoms to appear. For example, one boy, who was born by elective caesarean section, had a sudden collapse and required artificial ventilation. A diagnosis was made from a brainscan and ultrasound studies, which showed that bilateral intraventricular brain haemorrhage had occurred. The child developed respiratory distress due to hyaline membrane disease secondary to prematurity.

The brain haemorrhage may have been due to caesarean section or to prematurity and a concurrent infection. In other patients similar symptoms resulting from cerebral damage developed over periods ranging from 6 weeks, a few months, to even years after birth.

Prevalence of cerebral birth injury

It is difficult to estimate how many brain-injured children there are in China. When I went to the country hospital of Shandong province to investigate the treatment of brain injured children, and lectured to doctors at the health centre of the people's commune, the total number of brain injured children in the province was 26, out of a population of 500 000. However, I do not know how this figure compares with the number of healthy children in Shandong.

It is estimated by the Spastic Society of Victoria that there are approximately three cases of cerebral palsy for every 1000 live births in Australia.

CLINICAL MANIFESTATIONS

According to the topographical distribution of damaged areas in the brain, patients with cerebral birth injury may be identified as having one or other of the following disorders:
Monoplegia: One upper or lower limb is affected (see Fig. 4.1 lesion A).
Diplegia: Involvement of four limbs with the lower limb more affected than the upper limb (see Fig. 4.1. lesion B).
Triplegia: Involvement of three limbs.

Quadriplegia: Involvement of four limbs. Double hemiplegia is also used, meaning that the upper limbs are more affected than the lower limbs and that there may be a congenital suprabulbar palsy (see Fig. 4.1 lesion B or C both sides).
Hemiplegia: One side of the body is affected (see Fig. 4.1 lesion D).
Paraplegia: Involvement of both lower limbs (see Fig. 4.1 lesion E).

TYPES OF CEREBRAL PALSY

The types of involvement are spasticity, rigidity, athetosis or hypotonicity (atonia). However cerebral palsy rarely remains hypotonic. These floppy babies usually become spastic, athetoid or ataxic. Athetoid and ataxic children are mostly quadriplegic, occasionally a hemiathetoid child is encountered.

The main occurences are spasticity, athetosis and ataxia. However, these classifications are not clear cut. The predominant symptoms will determine which category a patient belongs to. Consequently the therapist may have to treat symptoms of one type of cerebral palsy in a patient classified as belonging to another type.

Spasticity

Hypertonus is most marked in antigravity muscles; it may involve spasticity or rigidity. Various factors influence spasticity: for example, rest, sleep, and relaxation reduce the degree of spasticity, while pain, stress, and anxiety increase spasticity. Changes in

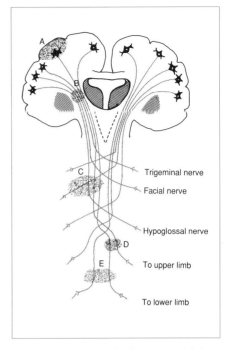

Fig. 4.1 Lesions in the pyramidal system. A. Lesion in the motor area of gyrus precentralis of the brain cortex; B. Lesion in the internal capsule; C. Lesion in one side of the pons; D. Lesion in one side of the cervical segment of the spinal cord; E. Transverse lesion in the thoracic segment of the spinal cord

hypertonus are seen with changes of position in some children; sudden movement, rather than slow movement, increases hypertonus. The tone in the plegic extremity can be modified by body position; tone in an affected upper limb, for example, is increased by turning the head away from it or by flexing the unaffected extremity against resistance. If spasticity creates pain during movement, it may also cause contractures.

Spasticity does not mean paralysis. Voluntary motion is present but may be laboured. Clinically, we often find if spasticity is decreased or removed by treatment, the spastic muscles may be strong, or slightly weak. The antagonist muscles may also be stronger after spasticity is decreased. Thus the function of the affected limb is restored to a level closer to normal.

The complications of spasticity are development of contractures of the joints and development of deformities of the limbs. Sometimes, spasticity may cause pain in the origins or insertions of spastic muscles. It may also lead to fractures.

Spasticity occurs often in patients with cerebral birth injury, but also in patients who have suffered brain damage (trauma, or after brain operations) and strokes. Sensory loss occasionally occurs in the spastic extremities.

Athetosis

Athetosis denotes continuous, slow or fast involuntary, arrhythmic movements that are always the same in the same patient and disappear during sleep. It may be uncontrollable and may impede voluntary movements that most commonly involve the distal segments of the limbs. They may be writhing, jerky, tremor, swiping, or rotary patterns or they may be unpatterned. Patients often perform the athetoid 'dance', unable to maintain weight on their feet, sometimes looking around and sometimes closing their eyes. Intelligence is good and may be high. The morbidity of athetosis is not high. In 300 clinical case histories we noted only 6 patients with athetosis (2%). In these, symptoms and signs were much improved after 3 months' treatment using acupressure therapy.

Ataxia

Ataxia is a clinical manifestation of cerebellar pathology characterised by disturbance of balance. The muscles contract irregularly and weakly. There is poor fixation of the head, trunk, shoulder and pelvic girdles. Tremor occurs when fine movements, such as buttoning clothes, writing, and shaving, are attempted. Muscle groups fail to work harmoniously and there is fragmentation of movement. Finger to finger, and finger to nose tests are a positive sign for the condition. A similar test can be performed on the lower limbs by asking the patient to place the heel of one foot on the shin of the opposite leg.

According to our observations, the ataxic case is relatively uncommon. At the Melbourne clinic we had 3 cases out of 30 patients with cerebral birth injury. (The ataxia was linked with cerebellar injury in these 3 cases.) This statistic (10%) also conforms to the incidence of ataxia at the Beijing Institute. Intelligence is often low, and patients can be clumsy and suffer multiple handicaps. Ataxic patients with signs and symptoms characteristic of pure ataxia are rare. Acupressure therapy for ataxic children is less effective than for patients presenting features of spastic and athetoid conditions.

◼ TREATMENT OF CEREBRAL BIRTH INJURY

Contraindications

The contraindications for treatment are as follows:

1. Acute diseases, for example, infections, acute abdominal diseases, suppurative arthritis, etc.
2. Severe heart disease, tuberculosis, malignant tumours
3. Haemorrhagic diseases, for example, haemophilia, purpura haemorrhagica, haemorrhagic glaucoma, haemorrhagic anaemia
4. Severe skin diseases
5. Poor general condition, for example, malnutrition, asthenia, collapse.

With cerebral birth injury, the younger the child is when beginning acupressure therapy, the better. Manipulations can start at 4 weeks of age. Adult patients with sequelae of cerebral birth injury can receive acupressure therapy, but there are many difficulties in treating adults and treatment may often not be successful.

What times or seasons are better for acupressure therapy in children? In our experience, the milder months are better for treatment: spring (3 months) and autumn (3 months). In winter, when the weather is cold, young children often catch cold, develop asthma, bronchitis, etc., after manipulation. During summer, if the weather is too hot, children may collapse, or suffer from heatstroke.

Table 4.2 Results of treatment in 30 cerebral birth injury patients

	Recovery	Improve-ment	No Change	Total
Mental retardation		14	4	18
Aphrenia			6	6
Aphasia		4	8	12
Dysphrasia	1	12	2	15
Cerebellar ataxia			4	4
Visual disturbance	1	20		21
Drooling	5	11	1	17
Opisthotonus	1	4		5
Epilepsy	1	10	1	12
Elevation of arm	15	4		19
Brush forehead with upper part of forearm	11	6		17
Touch opposite ear	17	7		24
Supination forearm	12	15		27
Touch spine with thumb	21	5		26
Difficulty in grasping	6	4		10
Inability to grasp	1	7	3	11
Inability to sit up	9	7	2	18
Inability to stand		27	1	28
Inability to walk		14	14	28
Scissor legs	11	4		15
Limp and sluggish gait	1	2	1	4
Abduction of hip joint	12	5		17
Internal rotation of thigh	24	3		27
External rotation of thigh	17	1		18
Stretch and elevation of leg	18	7		25
4-form test in prone position	20	6		26
Contracture of iliotibial tract	13			13
Allis' sign			1	1
Flexion contracture of knee joint	2	8		10
Drop foot	6	4		10
Equinovarus	1	3		4
Equinovalgus	6	5	1	12
Talipes calcaneus	1	2	1	4

Curative effect

At the end of each course of treatment, during the holiday period, I stay in my office, and sitting with my eyes closed, I think over the course, the results, and the curative effect of the treatment. How many cases have had a good result? How many patients have improved in their symptoms and signs? What is unsatisfactory?

My assistant and I consulted all of the 30 case histories of patients we treated in Melbourne to review our treatment. The following is a statistical analysis of results of treatment in patients with sequelae of cerebral birth injury (see Table 4.2 on previous page).There were 16 male and 14 female patients. Age distribution is shown in Table 4.3. The majority of the 30 patients were aged from 2 to 6 years.

Table 4.3 Age distribution of the 30 cerebral birth injury patients treated

							Total
Age (years)	2	3	4	5	6	8-14	
Number	5	8	8	4	3	2	30

The causes of cerebral birth injury in these 30 patients are shown in Table 4.4

Table 4.4 Causes of cerebral birth injury in the 30 patients treated

	Number
Premature delivery	14
Twins with difficult labour	2
Protracted labour with anoxia	11
Protracted labour with caesarean section	3
Total	30

• **Clinical diagnosis**

Some pathological changes were confirmed by ultrasound, CT scan, or laboratory test. There were 4 cases of intraventricular brain haemorrhage; 2 cases with hydrocephalus (the CT scan showed ventricle dilation due to aqueductual stenosis); and 2 patients with bacterial meningitis which possibly was connected with delivery. The types of clinical picture were spasticity in 26 cases; ataxia in 3 cases; and athetosis in 1 case. Topographically, of the 26 cases of spasticity there were 24 patients with quadriplegia and only 2 cases with hemiplegia. The number of sessions of treatment received by the patients is shown in Table 4.5

Table 4.5 Sessions of treatment received by the 30 patients

Sessions	Cases
20 to 30	1
31 to 40	3
41 to 50	4
61 to 70	20
more than 80	2
Total	30

• **Results of treatment**

From Table 4.2 it can be seen that the results of acupressure therapy differed according to the clinical situations.

• There were good results in recovery of function of the shoulders, hands, hip joints, and feet.
• For correction of scissor-legs, drop foot, equinovarus, equinovalgus, and contracture of iliotibial tract there were satisfactory results.
• Patients with visual problems obtained excellent curative results.

- Treatment of drooling, enuresis and constipation obtained good results.
- In the area of mental retardation, according to the parents' observations, there were some changes in the children, such as more interest in objects and in things around them. They responded faster to stimulation, sometimes with a smile. They seemed to understand more of what their parents were talking about, and some children became naughty, joined in games or conversed with others. Other children gradually began to understand what was on television shows and had an expression of happiness on their faces as they watched. Some took part in play with other children. Apart from noting such changes, the children's mental condition generally had little or no change after 3 months treatment, especially in severe cases. There were 4 patients with no change in their mental retardation in a total of 30 cases.
- There was some difference between children and adults regarding improvement with speech problems through treatment with acupressure therapy. The curative effect was limited in children, but was of much benefit to the adults who suffered with the effects of brain trauma and cerebrovascular accident.
- There were 12 cases of patients complicated with epilepsy. Treatment employed both acupressure therapy and the oral administration of antiepileptics, which were used before acupressure therapy and continued during the period of treatment. We found that in many cases the seizures decreased appreciably after 3 months treatment. And we also found that, in one case, seizures increased due to strong stimulation, but when treatment ceased, the seizure was decreased.

CASE HISTORY — *Male, aged 2 years*
First visit, 1 May 1989

The patient was born at 39 weeks, and was small for full term. He was underweight for a 2-year old (5500 g). His mother reported that he was very active during pregnancy. He kept turning and the placenta was good, but the umbilical cord was twisted like a telephone cord, and he was anoxic as a result of lack of adequate blood supply prenatally. An emergency caesarian section was done at 39 weeks of pregnancy. The fetal heart monitor prior to birth showed that he was in distress. After the birth, he was put into a humidicrib for a few hours; later he started having seizures and going blue. The fits could not be stabilized so he was flown by air ambulance to a metropolitan hospital. He was put on carbamazepine and phenobarbitone medication. Cerebral palsy with epilepsy and damage to the frontal lobe of the brain was diagnosed. The patient had a regular physiotherapy programme before Chinese acupressure therapy.

• Acupressure treatment

The patient had 43 sessions of treatment at the Melbourne clinic. This was carried out daily five times a week from 1 May 1989 to 6 July 1989. The treatment was directed at drooling, and vision in both eyes, and included manipulation for the two shoulder joints and forearms, and both hands. We also concentrated on sitting, standing and walking. Orthopaedic manipulations combined with percussion, pressing points, etc. were applied to both hip joints, knee joints, and ankle joints and feet to relax the spastic muscles, and correct the deformities and scissor-legs. Epilepsy was treated by pressing of antiepileptic points in addition to the use of antiepileptics. When mild manipulation was given, the fits occurred less frequently; after strong stimulation, however, the fitting was worse.

Flexion contracture of both knee joints was corrected by the use of manipulations (see Fig. 3.25) and external fixation (see Fig. 3.55). Results of treatment were satisfactory (see Table 4.6 on next page).

Further treatment and exercises at home were suggested as follows:

1. Continuing the movement of shoulder and hip joints
2. Continuing the splints and manipulations for correction of flexion contracture of the knee joints
3. Continuing the treatment of epilepsy
4. Speech exercises
5. Standing and walking exercises.

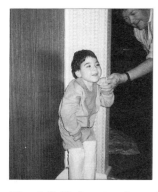

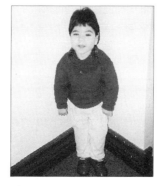

Fig. 4.2 Before treatment

Fig. 4.3 After 43 sessions of treatment

Table 4.6 Results of treatment - Male, aged 2 years

Before treatment	After treatment
1. Range of movement in shoulder joints	
Elevation of arms limited to 90° passively	Elevation of arms reached to 180° passively
Could not touch the spine passively with either thumb	Could touch spine using right and left thumb passively
2. Limitation of supination of forearms in both sides	In both forearms supination was normal in range
3. Unable to sit up	Sat independently
4. Stood with support	Stood against a corner
5. Inability to walk	No change
6. Functional disturbance in hip joints Abducted hip joints to 30 cm between the inner borders of the two patellae	Abducted the hip joints to 45 cm (normal range)
Internal and external rotation limited	Internal and external rotation were normal in range
Stretch and elevation of legs limited to 45° on both sides	Stretch and elevation of legs reached 90° (normal range)
4-form test positive in prone position, indicating that contractures of Rectus femoris and Iliopsoas were present. Consequently, had a forward tilted pelvis.	4-form test negative, in prone position. The pelvic tilt had disappeared, the waist straightened.
Ober's sign positive on both sides indicating that contractures of both iliotibial tracts were present	Ober's sign negative on both sides
7. Flexion contracture of the knee joints	Flexion contracture of the knee joints corrected
8. Drop foot on both sides	Drop foot on both sides corrected
9. Scissor-legs	Scissor-legs corrected
10. Visual problems. Strabismus and shortsight	Visual problems improved

CASE HISTORY — *Male, aged 4 years 6 months*

The patient's complaints were impaired function of the four limbs and vision, and no speech, following cerebral damage due to meningitis in the early neonatal period.

The patient was born prematurely at 31 weeks, and developed meningitis followed by hydrocephalus. He had a shunt (subcutaneous ventriculoperitoneal on the right side). At 12 months he was diagnosed as having cerebral palsy with severe visual defect with some degree of optic atrophy. His legs were more affected than his arms, and the right side more affected than the left.

He had developmental delay in mental condition. In the previous 2 years, he had received conductive education, physiotherapy, and treatment at a school for blind children, and his mother had worked with him using hot baths and warm up exercises to relax his muscles before he practised walking guided by a ladder-back chair or by his mother's hands. He made good progress but continued to be severely multiply disabled. He sat independently. He used his hands for feeding, and drank from a cup by himself. He crawled everywhere and liked to explore. He also liked to stand and walk with assistance but his legs crossed. He pulled himself to standing and could side step around a bench, holding on with his hands. His vision was very selective but improving. He used sign language with his hands to indicate his basic needs: sleep, food, drink, toilet, 'more' and 'no more'. He had a sense of humour and liked to be naughty in his own small way. He was a happy, good natured child.

On 26 January 1989 he had his first visit to the Chinese acupressure therapy clinic in Melbourne. After assessment we made a diagnosis of quadriplegia, visual disturbance, and aphasia resulting from the postnatal cerebral injury. The positive clinical findings are recorded in Table 4.7 on the next page. To enable a comparison to be made of symptoms and signs before and after treatment, the results of therapy are included also in the Table.

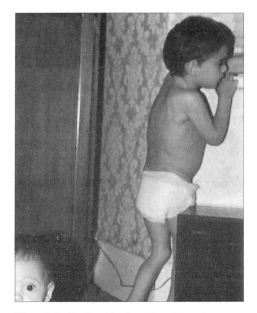

Fig. 4.4 Patient before treatment

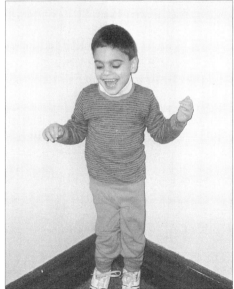

Fig. 4.5 Patient after treatment

Table 4.7 Results of treatment - Male, aged 4 years 6 months

Before treatment	After treatment
1. Mental condition	
Sensory-motor understanding estimated at 8 - 10 months (based on sighted norms)	Sensory-motor understanding estimated at 12 - 18 months level (some gaps; based on sighted norms)
	Beginning imaginative play; improved concentration; improved co-operation and interaction with other people
2. Visual condition	
Use of vision appeared to be fleeting and inconsistent. Patient made eye contact but did not maintain it. His visual attention was mostly in response to sound cues, when he would look briefly at an object and then look away	Eyes more alive and expressive, uses vision well for mobility, tracking, distance and location of judging size, approximate objects; has no field losses; eye contact greatly improved, can make eye contact through peep holes at 1 m in very dim light
Optic atrophy, strong autistic avoidance pattern	Still prefers to use touch to find objects. Forgets to look. Not yet looking and doing at the same time. This is typical of optic atrophy
3. Speech problems	
He said 'yeah' for 'yes' and shook his head for 'no'. He used sign language with his hands. Communication was non-verbal	Improved receptive and expressive language, follows unrelated commands, more vocal and with more meaning 'go car, go bath, ca (cat), up, good boy, go out Uses voice synthesizer unit to express food and drink choices
4. Functional movements in the shoulder joint. Touching spine with the thumb was limited on both sides	Touching spine with thumb free on both sides
5. Supination of forearm limited	Supination of forearm free on right side, improved on left side
6. Able to stand up from being seated on his stool, he was able to bear all his weight, but required holding	Able to stand up from being seated on his stool without any assistance or holding
7. Walked with two handed support, legs crossed. Trunk flexed, muscle tone increased in legs	Walks with frame support. A little cross-legged. His little cross-legged. His walking with frame support and the spastic muscles are obviously relaxed, but the gait is not a normal pattern

Table 4.7 Results of treatment - Male, aged 4 years 6 months cont.

Before treatment	After treatment
8. Hip joints	
Abduction of the hip joints limited to 34 cm between the two inner borders of the patellas	Abduction of the hip joints now reaches 50 cm
Both internal and external rotation of hip joints limited	External and internal rotation correct to the normal range
Stretch and elevation of legs limited	Stretch and elevation of legs reaches normal range
4-form test positive in prone	4-form test negative
Ober's sign positive in right side	Ober's sign negative

CASE HISTORY — Male, aged 6 years

The patient visited our clinic in Nanfen in 1987 and 1988. He was born after the normal period of gestation and suffered anoxia in the uterus due to early rupture of the amnion and delayed birth. The baby weighed 3.5 kilograms at birth, when he was seen to be cyanotic and in respiratory distress. He received emergency treatment for a few hours and recovered. When he was 8 months old, his parents found that he could not sit or crawl, had a weak neck and spinal column, had difficulty raising his head, and had muscle stiffness in all four limbs. At that time, he had no speech. At the age of 3 years, however, he began to speak but was dysphasic.

He was examined in the county hospital, Wuhan, and Shanghai Shu-guang Hospital and he was given drugs, massage, and acupuncture treatment with no satisfactory results.

In July 1987, he came to the acupressure clinic of Nanfen for treatment. Clinical examination showed limitation of movement in both shoulder joints, for example in elevating the arms, touching the opposite ear, and touching the spine with the thumb. Supination of the forearms was also limited. He had difficulty in grasping in both hands, he could sit but could not stand or walk independently. Movement in his hip joints was also limited as demonstrated by the usual methods of evaluating hip joint function such as internal and external rotation, abduction of the joint, elevation of the legs, and the 4-form test on the legs. He had drop foot on both sides.

Routine treatment for cerebral palsy was given, selecting the points of the head, face and limbs, and correcting the deformities by the use of orthopaedic manipulation. The treatment was carried out once daily for 12 weeks, and then for another 2 months after a gap of 6 months. The results of treatment were that movement in both shoulder joints reached normal range, and the patient was then able to feed himself. There was also great improvement in the function of both hip joints, so that he could now stand and walk without assistance. Figures 4.6 and 4.7 on the next page show the patient before and after treatment

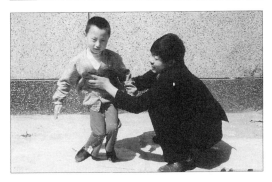

Fig. 4.6 Male patient aged 6, who suffered with cerebral palsy, before treatment, standing with support

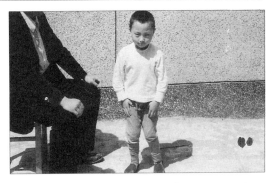

Fig. 4.7 Patient after 5 months treatment standing independently

CASE HISTORY — *Female, aged 5 years*
Date of birth, 9 March 1984.

In March 1989 the patient made her first visit to the acupressure clinic in Melbourne. Her chief complaints were multiple functional disabilities for 5 years due to cerebral birth injury. The patient was 22 weeks premature delivered with Neville-Barnes forceps. Her birth weight was 664 g. She was incubated for a period of 2 months in total. Her initial problem was hyaline membrane disease of moderate severity, requiring ventilation. The initial recovery period was complicated by a pneumothorax and mild pulmonary haemorrhage. She developed a multi resistant Staphylococcus aureus (MRSA) pneumonia that complicated her ventilatory therapy at about one month of age, and at that time she required increasing ventilatory support.

She had bilateral ventricular haemorrhages that were present on the third day and grade 3 in severity. Follow-up scans showed some extension of the haemorrhages into the cortical regions, accompanied by only mild dilation of the ventricles. Fourteen days after birth she developed convulsions. Investigations at that stage showed the presence of MRSA in her cerebrospinal fluid.

Treatment with chloramphenicol and vancomycin was given and continued for a period of 6 weeks. Head scans showed the development of porencephaly in association with the meningitis. The ultrasound report prior to her discharge was summarized as saying 'The outline of the left lateral ventricle is irregular and there is a 6 mm porencephalic cyst present just above the ventricle. Intraventricular adhesions are present anteriorly.' There was probably also an area of porencephaly anterior to the frontal horn. Her convulsions were reasonably well controlled with phenobarbitone and phenytoin and she was discharged from hospital on phenobarbitone. A diagnosis of blindness was also made. The neurological deficit was the consequence of the bilateral intraventricular haemorrhages and meningitis. She returned home on 14 September 1984.

• Acupressure treatment

When this patient came to the acupressure therapy clinic for treatment in March 1989, her general condition was not good; she was weak, tired, and had no interest in anything. Spasticity of arms and legs was evident, and she had intermittent convulsions. The clinical findings before and after treatment for 3 months (81 sessions) are set out in Table 4.8.

Table 4.8 Result of treatment

Before treatment	After treatment
1. Mental retardation	Improved
2. Aphasia	No change
3. Drooling	Stopped
4. Shoulder joint motion limited	Free passive shoulder joint motion
5. Supination of forearm limited on both sides	Improved on both sides
6. Unable to grasp	No change
7. Unable to sit up	Sits with support
8. Unable to stand	No change
9. Unable to walk	No change
10. Abduction of hip joint, 18 cm	Increased to 25 cm (normal range)
11. Limited internal rotation of hip joint both sides	Normal range on both sides
12. Limited external rotation of hip joint both sides	Normal range both sides
13. 4-form test positive in prone position	Normal range both sides
14. Bilateral visual defects	Improved both sides
15. Scissor-leg	Corrected
16. Convulsions	Rare
17. Poor appetite	Appetite improved
18. General condition bad. Crying feeble	General conditon good, cried loudly
19. A lot of spasm in back muscles and muscles of all four limbs	All muscles relaxed

CASE HISTORY — Female, aged 2 years 6 months

The patient was the first born of twins by caesarian section on 16 August 1986. At 5 weeks after birth, she developed bronchitis producing a high temperature and respiratory failure. She was intubated and ventilated and sent to an intensive care unit. At this time her parents were warned that brain damage (cerebral palsy) was possible and it was later confirmed. The patient attended physiotherapy sessions at the hospital for an hour and a half weekly. The parents also contacted the intellectual disability services, which arranged fortnightly visits to her home by a speech pathologist and an occupational therapist. 'This was a very frustrating time for us, as she was not making very much progress; she was very tight and could do nothing at all. It would take up to an hour or more just to feed her one meal' her mother said.

In June 1987 when she was 12 months old her parents made contact with a national centre and started an intensive programme of therapy at home. Some of the exercises were patterning, hip stretching, hanging upside down, and using a torch to help increase vision along with many others. This therapy programme continued for a year and a half. About that time, microcephaly, epilepsy, and a winged scapula on the right shoulder were diagnosed.

Six months after starting this therapeutic programme, she began regular visits to a chiropractor. 'With all the therapy we were giving her we found that she started to improve' said her parents. 'Her vision improved, she started moving her legs and it was getting easier to feed her'. She started to take notice of things around her and began to respond when her parents talked to her. 'Before we started this therapy programme, she had severe squints in both eyes. They slowly started to go away' her parents said. 'It didn't matter what we tried we could not get rid of the spasticity. Her arms did not seem to get much better either. We worked hard with our daughter, we also kept looking for other things to help her.'

In January 1989 this patient began treatment at the Chinese acupressure therapy clinic in Melbourne. The following positive clinical findings were noted and these formed the basis of her treatment with acupressure and therapeutic manipulation. Clinical examination showed inability to sit, stand or walk. She had no speech, and there were visual problems in both eyes, and a long term condition of drooling. Her right shoulder movements were limited, as in touching the opposite ear, touching her spine with her thumb, etc. Supination of the forearm was limited on the right side. There was inability to grasp with either hand. Her hip joint movement was limited in both internal and external rotation. The stretch and elevation of her legs was 60° on both sides. The 4-form test of the legs in prone position was positive on both sides. She had drop foot on both sides and crossed legs during walking when supported with two hands. Abduction of the hip joint was limited; the distance between the two inner borders of the patella was 21 cm (see Fig. 4.8).

She received acupressure therapy daily from January to April 1989, 60 sessions in total. After she started acupressure therapy there was a great change in her and her father said: 'Everything we have tried to achieve with other therapies - and did not succeed with - has shown us just how much acupressure has helped our daughter.'

Her spasticity had been reduced so much she now had a full range movements of arms and legs. For the first time in 2 years 6 months she could cross her legs and began to learn to sit on the floor using her arms for balance (see Fig. 4.9). She was so much more aware of the things around her, her reaching improved and also her speech. She could say 'hungry', 'love you', 'Mummy', etc. Her general condition, sleep, and appetite were better than they were before treatment. She had stopped drooling. There was a lot of improvement of vision in both eyes and she could watch an object and respond to sound stimulation and light. Drop feet and cross legs were corrected, the hip joints could expand within normal range. Her father said, 'The list goes on, we know we still have a long way to go but the road seems so much brighter now. Again I must say acupressure therapy was a major step in her life. It has given us hope we never had before. One day our daughter is going to stand and walk.'

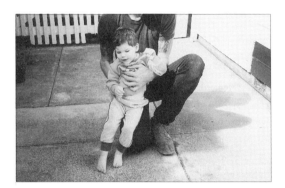

Fig. 4.8 Before treatment

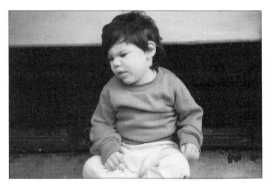

Fig. 4.9 Patient after 3 months treatment. She can sit well and is doing exercises to facilitate standing and walking

CASE HISTORY — Male, aged 6 years 6 months
Date of birth, 22 July 1982

The patient was born 13 weeks premature after a difficult delivery through the birth canal with obstetric forceps. His birth weight was 1220 g. He was ventilated for 10 days, during which time he suffered many episodes of apnoea as well as a respiratory collapse. He spent 8 weeks in oxygen and had continued episodes of apnoea. A further 8 weeks was spent in nursery care at the hospital prior to being released into parent care. His mother noticed that at the age of 8 months, he would kick only with the left leg, and reach only with the left arm. He was diagnosed at the time as having cerebral palsy with a right hemiplegia. Care was provided in the first instance by a hospital growth and development clinic. A CT scan was carried out to check cerebral damage including the speech area of the cerebral cortex. He was referred at the age of 2 years for intensive speech therapy. His physiotherapy and occupational therapy were ongoing.

In his medical history, it was reported that he was independently mobile but had decreased awareness of the right side. There was also involuntary muscle tone and some weakness in muscle groups of the right side. These factors led to a tendency for him to have his right arm in a fixed position during gross and fine motor activities, such as writing, jumping and running. His body rotated slightly causing him to leave his right leg behind, and lessened his performance in higher level activities such as jumping and running.

In May 1989 the patient attended the Chinese acupressure therapy clinic in Melbourne for treatment.

Clinical findings before and after treatment are described below. The clinical findings before acupressure treatment:

- Movement at the right shoulder joint was limited in touching his left ear with the right hand; and limited in touching his spine with the right thumb.
- Supination of right forearm was limited.
- Abduction and extension movements of the right thumb were limited. Opposition of the right thumb to the right index, middle, ring and small fingers was not possible so that the patient could not pick up small objects with his right hand. Grasp in the right hand was weaker than that of the left hand and the patient could not make a full fist due to claw fingers in the right hand.
- The hip joint was limited in internal rotation. The 4-form test in prone position (see Fig. 3.22) was positive (meaning that his right Rectus femoris and Iliopsoas muscles were contracted.) This led to limited motor activities, such as in walking and running. Contracture of the iliotibial tract on the right side, resulted in abduction deformity of the hip joint during walking and running.
- As to the ankle joint, there was equinovarus on the right side, and limited dorsiflexion of the right foot.
- As to gross motor activites, the patient walked with a limp and a slight sluggish gait, the right foot dropped and moved in a circular motion, and the right elbow was flexed and had a fixed posture during gross motor activities.

The acupressure treatment was carried out once daily, involving the following manipulations and exercises:

- Manipulation of the right shoulder joint to touch left ear with right hand (see Fig. 3.5) to touch spine with right thumb (see Fig. 3.6).
- Rotation of the right forearm with a backward movement (see Fig. 3.7) 20-30 times for one treatment.
- Manipulation on the right hand to correct the deformities of the thumb and fingers, in addition to the use of a splint (see Fig. 3.10) and physical exercise such as grasping, making a fist, picking up coins, holding a pen and writing (see Fig. 3.13).

Treatment for the right lower extremity was also given once every day. This involved internal rotation of the right hip joint (see Fig. 3.17), the 4-form test in prone position on both sides (see Fig. 3.22) and manipulation for correction of contracture of the iliotibial tract (see Figs 3.20, 3.21) and equinovarus. At the same time we asked him to do exercises at home, such as standing, jumping, and hopping on his right foot and running.

The results of 40 sessions of treatment given over 2 months were as follows. The patient had progressed well in the gross motor area. He walked and ran without a limp or sluggish gait. His equinovarus had been corrected, and he could jump without support. He moved his right arm while walking. He had reasonable voluntary control over his right arm and hand. He was able to open his fingers on command and make a fist normally. He could pick up coins from the ground and put them into a box. His writing was illegible before treatment but became neat and legible after treatment. Abduction of the right thumb was within normal range but upward movement of the thumb on command was still a little limited. There was normal range of movement in the right shoulder, elbow and wrist joints. Independence in all activities would be encouraged, but the patient still needed a little assistance in some areas, tying shoe laces, tying knots, etc.

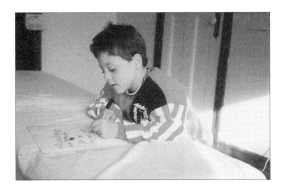

Fig. 4.10 Patient before treatment

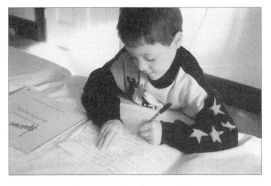

Fig. 4.11 Patient after 10 weeks treatment

CASE HISTORY — *Female, aged 3 years 6 months*
Date of birth, 12 April 1985

The patient's first visit to the Chinese acupressure clinic in Melbourne was in January 1989. Her chief complaint was major neurological and developmental problems over the previous 3 years.

The patient was born following a normal pregnancy and delivery. She was found apnoeic and cyanotic in her cot 14 days after birth. She was resuscitated by her mother, taken to a district hospital in severe respiratory distress, and intubated. She was treated with intravenous ampicillin and gentamicin and transferred to a children's hospital. On arrival she was ventilated, and had several seizures requiring phenobarbitone, phenytoin, diazepam, and clonazepam, but these had ceased by 30 May 1985, by which time she was on phenobarbitone alone. The first seizure was on 28 May 1985 followed by three further episodes. A head ultrasound performed that day showed 'the ventricular system appeared small with mild increase of periventricular white matter echogenicity; the sulci appeared echogenic. The finding is suggestive of cerebral oedema and subarachnoid haemorrhage'. Endoscopy performed on 30 May 1985 revealed mild swelling of the vocal cord secondary to the presence of the endotracheal tube. On 31 May 1985 head ultra-sound again showed evidence of oedema. Phenytoin was withdrawn and the administration of phenobarbitone was changed from the intravenous to the oral form. Chest X-ray showed right upper lobe collapse.

The patient remained intubated and ventilated. By 2 June 1985 she was extubated and put on headbox oxygen and, after showing some improvement, was returned to atmospheric respiration on 3 June 1985. Clinical assessment at the time showed increased tone in the upper limbs and decreased tone in the lower limbs, placing but no stepping, good grasp, and poor head control. The EEG showed multiple epileptiform activity. The final diagnosis at the children's hospital was hypoxia-induced convulsions and cerebral damage. Treatment on discharge: phenobarbitone 10.5 mg twice daily. She was again admitted to the district hospital on 29 November 1986 with repeated minor convulsions, which were not being controlled in the home setting. These convulsions were observed in hospital and consisted mainly of sudden disturbance in conscious state associated with slight hyperextension of the body and head, with stiffening and trembling of the upper limbs, and sometimes eye deviation to the left. They were only of 5-10 seconds duration but occurred many times in the course of an hour. She was treated by oral high dose prednisolone, a single daily dose of 20 mg in the morning, adding clonazepam 0.5 mg also as a morning dose, in addition to her regular sodium valproate and carbamazepine. Over the couple of days in hospital, the frequency of the seizures dropped, and she was discharged home on sodium valproate 5 ml (200 mg) twice a day, carbamazepine 100 mg twice a day, and clonazepam 0.5 mg in the morning. Her fits were steroid responsive and she was treated with prednisolone 20 mg per day for 6 weeks (4 December 86 to 20 January 87). She was then changed to frisium (clobazam) 10 mg twice a day, with carbamazepine 100 mg with a reducing dose of prednisolone, to cease in about 4 to 5 weeks time. Prednisolone for 6 weeks was not successful, but with the frisium the seizure activity reduced. This was used in combination with sodium valproate, after gradual withdrawal of carbamazepine.

The patient's medical history records that on 1 August 1987 she had been very heavily sedated for a long time but was still having quite a number of small fits. She could turn her eyes to locate sounds and was functioning at about a 5 - 6-month-old level.

On 19 February 1988 she was seen to be more alert and responsive, but was still having many fits. Her receptive language levels were low. Before our Chinese acupressure therapy, she was under the care of a paediatrician and the State spastic society. She had a diagnosis of cortical blindness (light perception only).

• Acupressure treatment

The patient had 2 courses of Chinese acupressure treatment at the Melbourne clinic starting in January 1989. This was carried out by me once daily for 3 months. There was a gap of 4 weeks, followed by the second course, from May 1989 June 1989. The patient had altogether 83 sessions of acupressure treatment. The manipulations were applied as routine techniques of acupressure therapy on the eyes, hands, shoulders, arms, lower limbs, including manipulation for drooling, etc. Table 4.9 on the next page shows the results of treatment.

We suggested the family contact the clinic in the future for consultation and further suggestions for exercises or treatment, and that in the meantime, the family continue to do manipulation and exercises at home.

Table 4.9 Results of 83 sessions of treatment - Female aged 3 years 6 months

Before treatment	After treatment
1. Mental retardation	Improved
2. Aphasia	Improved
3. Visual problems	Much improved
4. Drooling	Ceased
5. Shoulder movements limited in elevation of arms, touching opposite ear, touching spine with thumb	All movements in both shoulder joints normal
6. Supination of forearm limited on both sides	Supination of both forearms in normal range
7. Difficulty in grasping both sides	Able to grasp with both hands
8. Unable to sit up	Able to sit
9. Unable to stand	Able to stand with support
10. Unable to walk	Able to walk with support
11. Abducted hip joint with difficulty	Normal range of movement, no pain
12. Internal and external rotation of hip joint limited	Normal range of movement
13. Stretch and elevate legs 70° passively	Increased to 80° in both legs
14. 4-form test of legs in prone position positive on both sides	Normal
15. Iliotibial tract contracture on both sides	Corrected both sides
16. Flexion contracture of both knee joints	Both knee joints relaxed after manipulation and splinting
17. Epilepsy seizure a few times daily	Ceased

CASE HISTORY — *Male, aged 6 years*

The patient was born 6 weeks premature and had breathing problems. He suffered a haemorrhage in the brain 1 week after birth. He was shown to have bilateral intraventricular brain haemorrhage as diagnosed by ultrasound. He was diagnosed as having spastic quadriplegia and intellectual impairment. He could not stand or walk unaided as his leg muscles were severely spastic. He was already showing delayed development of speech. He also had a squint for which he attended an eye clinic with a view to operative correction. It was believed that his visual acuity was within normal limits.

Clinical examination in January 1989 showed the patient had dysphasia, drooling, and limited movements in the shoulder joints. He could not touch the opposite ear with his fingers, and he could not touch his spine with his thumb. Supination of the forearm behind the head was limited. He had difficulty grasping in both hands. He was unable to stand or walk. He had contracture of the hip abductors. Internal and external rotation of the hip joints were limited. Stretch and elevation of the legs was to 60°. The 4-form test of legs in prone position was positive on both sides. He had drop foot on both sides. His right and left knee joints were contracted in about 20° of flexion. He walked with support exhibiting a scissor gait (see Fig. 4.12).

The patient attended the acupressure therapy clinic in Melbourne, where he received daily acupressure therapy and some orthopaedic manipulations. He also had intermittant fixation with splints for a period of 3 months. He received 63 sessions of treatment in the 3 months.

Results of treatment were determined on 7 April 1989. The drooling had stopped; but there was no change in his dysphasia. There was normal range of movement in both shoulder joints; supination of both forearms was much improved; and grasping in both hands was also improved. There was normal range of movement of the hip joints in all directions; stretch and elevation of the legs was 90°. The 4-form test was negative on both sides; and the drop foot, scissor legs and flexion contracture of the knee joints were almost completely corrected. The patient could stand and walk with the support of a walking frame or a chair (see Fig. 4.13). In April 1989 he began to attend normal school.

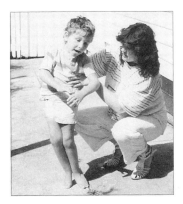

Fig. 4.12 Patient before treatment standing with the support of two hands

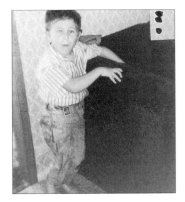

Fig. 4.13 Patient in standing position after 63 sessions of therapy

CHAPTER 5

HEAD INJURY AND BRAIN DAMAGE

Head injury constitutes a major health problem in all nations. Reports that include all patients with head injuries (irrespective of severity) within a defined population are not readily available, and the descriptive elements of the epidemiology are therefore incomplete. There are many causes of head injury, including road accidents, assault, falls, domestic, sport/leisure, work/school accidents, etc. Strang et al (1978) have reported on the causes of head injury by age group (see Table 5.1).

Table 5.1 Causes of head injury by age group

Cause	Age		
	under 15 yr	15-64 yr	over 65 yr
		%	
Road accidents	9	24	24
Assault	3	24	1
Falls	16	13	28
Domestic	27	8	29
Sport/leisure	21	6	1
Work/school	4	12	2

As time goes on and with the steady growth of motorcar production, I believe that the number of road accidents and head injuries will also increase in all countries of the world. Currently, the numbers affected are considerable. Figures vary but range from some 8 severely brain injured people per 100 000 population to 150 with severe resultant disability per 100 000 population. Head injury has been referred to as a silent epidemic. In the United States there are said to be 40 times as many head injuries each year as spinal cord injuries.

In Australia, the National Head Injury Foundation has estimated that each year, between 50 000 and 90 000 people suffer head injury. Two-thirds of these people are below the age of 30. The Australian Brain Foundation reports that every year more than 40 000 Australians of all ages are admitted to hospital with some kind of head injury.

Pathological changes as a result of brain injury

Head injury pathology makes a distinction between impact and secondary brain damage. Impact damage includes fracture of the skull, contusions of the grey matter and diffuse lesions of the white matter. Secondary brain damage includes intracranial haematoma and ischaemic brain damage and is associated with raised intracranial pressure.

There is a pathological basis for the late effects of head injury. Residual disability or newly developing complications (epilepsy or hydrocephalus) may be related to impact damage, to the serious early secondary pathological processes, or to later events such as scarring or adhesions causing traction on parts of the brain or blockage of cerebrospinal fluid pathways.

Irreversible brain damage in some patients has proven to be not the result of severe impact damage, but a consequence of resusciation following cardio-respiratory arrest. Clinically, post-traumatic dementia, cerebral hemisphere dysfunction, hemiplegia, hemianopia, and dysphasia are common sequelae of severe injury.

Hydrocephalus is often found in cases with extensive diffuse brain damage, and is sometimes seen after a focal lesion such as an intracerebral haematoma. Obstructive hydrocephalus is often found in sub-arachnoid haemorrhage, and adhesions from this cause may lead to blockage in various parts of cerebrospinal fluid circulation. Post-traumatic epilepsy is caused by scars produced by cortical damage, in cases of depressed fracture or diffuse damage.

Clinical features persisting after brain damage are as follows: headache; dizziness; facial paralysis; dribbling; dysfunction of speech; visual problems; hemiplegia; quadriplegia; paraplegia; dysfunction and deformities of wrist and hands; dysfunction and deformities of hip, knee and ankle joints, and foot; defective control of micturition and defecation; constipation; and epilepsy.

Differences between children and adults when considering treatment following head injury or cerebral damage are listed in Table 5.2.

Table 5.2 Differences in treatment of children and adults

	Children	Adults
Likelihood of fractures	Less likely	More likely (e.g., neck of femur or humerus)
Range of joint movements	Full	Stop before going too far
Frequency of treatment	Daily or every other day	Every other day or, rarely, every day
Intensity of stimulation	Mild, medium, less use of strong	Medium, more use of strong, mild, medium for the elderly
Recovery	Early with quick improvement	Late and sometimes slow
Approach to functional exercises	Initial emphasis on passive movement	Patients encouraged to do exercises on own initiative (active)

◼ TREATMENT OF HEAD INJURY

The needs of brain damaged people are great. Advances in medical technology play an ever-increasing and important part, especially in the acute and comatose stages. There is also a high cost in terms of human resources, which diminishes only when the patients are discharged.

Management in the acute stage

All head injuries require an initial assessment of the type of injury sustained, for example, diffuse or focal, mild or severe, open or closed, and with or without extracranial injuries or complications. All patients have then to be monitored for the onset of developing complications that may call for treatment. A minority will need an operation, for example, when there are open injuries or because an intracranial haematoma develops. In the management of milder injuries, opinions may differ about how closely, and for how long, patients need to be observed, and whether or not they require admission to hospital.

In the case of the patient with head injury who is in coma, there are two major needs before admission to hospital: (a) maintenance of an effective airway; and (b) monitoring of responsiveness. The response to these needs varies widely. In some places it has been possible to organize mobile intensive care units, staffed by highly trained personnel. In Beijing there is an efficient emergency communication system linking the Institute of Neurology in Tiantan Hospital to the county or district, and people's village hospitals. Emergency services can be called on through the telephone. A first aid team of specialists in acute brain damage care can be called to any local hospital fully equipped for emergency care, and even head operations. Acute cases can be transferred by this team to the Institute of Neurology for further treatment if necessary, once their condition is stable. This greatly reduces mortality from brain damage.

Primary care of mild brain injuries, for the talking and walking patient, involves initial assessment of central nervous system signs and examination for other injuries. Three measures may then be necessary: repair of any scalp wound, skull radiography, and continuing observation. All patients who are unconscious run the risk of respiratory obstruction. There are the additional risks of hypoxia, hypotension, and other systemic events that can harm the recently damaged brain. Comatose cases must be afforded the care proper to this stage and attention to the head injury itself initially takes second place to ensuring that the body is well perfused with adequately oxygenated blood. After head injury, the patient risks partial obstruction of the airway perhaps due to the tongue falling backwards, aspiration of vomitus, blood, secretions, foreign bodies or CSF (cerebrospinal fluid). The risk begins at the roadside and continues during transport in the ambulance, in the accident and emergency department, the radiology department, the corridors and the elevators of the hospital, and even in the ward. Ten years ago most patients in coma after head injury had a tracheostomy, often performed soon after injury.

Hypotension may have disastrous effects upon a recently injured brain but is very rarely a consequence of injury to the brain.

Profuse haemorrhage from a scalp wound is rarely cause for concern, but injury from a major venous sinus can be serious. My experience as young doctor, fresh out of medical school, taught me very early that the use of clamps in treating head injuries was not recommended. This occurred when I was present during an operation on a patient who had a puncture wound from a 5 cm long steel nail. When the senior doctor performing the operation took out the nail, there was profuse haemorrhage from the superior sagittal sinus. The preferred technique for treatment at this stage was putting gauze into the wound and waiting for 10 minutes until the haemorrhage stopped. It was then possible to continue the operation, clean out the foreign bodies, and suture the wound. In this case the patient's condition was good and the operation was a success.

General medical care

After injury there is retention of salt and water and excretion of potassium. There is greater retention of water than sodium, resulting in mild hyponatremia, but this does not indicate a deficit of total body sodium. Another factor is redistribution of blood between the cortex and medulla of the kidney. This may be exacerbated by circulatory abnormalities.

In the first 3 or 4 days after head injury, fluid is best given intravenously as a dextrose/saline combination. For the adult, an intake of between 1500 to 2000 ml every 24 hours is necessary. If the patient remains in coma, the nasogastric route should be employed. The need to supply a more substantial amount of calories and other food sources will become important.

In nutrition of the injured patient who has a head injury only, the total energy requirements may be little different from normal. When starting nasogastric feeding, it has been my custom to use a combination of milk and water, 30 to 100 ml/hour. Where there are multiple injuries, it is probably sufficient to supply 2000 to 3000 calories per day. General medical care includes some other important aspects. The eyelids may need to be taped closed and lubricated periodically to prevent corneal damage from abrasion or dehydration. In order to prevent contractions of the joints the limbs should be put through as full a range of movements as possible several times a day. The immobilized patient needs to be turned every 2 hours and his skin rubbed and protected against pressure sores. Chest physiotherapy, in combination with posture drainage is important. The urinary bladder will usually empty reflexly.

ACUPRESSURE THERAPY

Recovery of function after acute brain damage is a remarkable phenomenon. The therapist should carefully study standardized methods available to measure changes in performance over time, so that recovery curves can be constructed for different functions. Recovery curves can provide a basis for distinguishing between spontaneous recovery and the results of therapy and thus are valuable in assessing the role of specific methods of rehabilitation. For example, after brain damage a boy with adduction contraction in both hip joints for 2 years received physiotherapy and conductive education for 18 months. At the first visit for acupressure therapy and manipulation, the distance between the medial margins of the two patellae was 20 cm. He received manipulation to abduct the hip joints once daily. After 10 sessions of treatment, the distance was 25 cm, after 15 sessions, 30 cm, and after 30 sessions, 39 cm, which is within the normal range of abduction of the hip joints in a boy of his height. It is clear that recovery of movement in the hip joints was the result of therapy and was not spontaneous.

Contraindications

The contraindications of acupressure therapy in patients after brain injuries are as follows:

1. Severe heart disease, tuberculosis, and malignant tumours
2. Poor general condition, such as weakness, poor appetite and sleep, and hypotension
3. Pregnancy and menstruation
4. Severe skin diseases
5. Haemorrhagic diseases.

CASE HISTORY — *Male, aged 22 years*

The patient was single, a student, with functional disturbance of the left arm and leg after a car accident 3 years before. After drinking with his friends one evening, he ran off the road driving home, and the car rolled several times. He was thrown from the car, and when the ambulance arrived at the scene, he was found unconscious. On arrival at the casualty department his blood pressure was 110/70 mmHg, the pulse rate was 70/min and regular and the respiratory rate 18/min. Examination of his central nervous system showed a right upwards gaze and some non-purposeful movement. He had both direct and consensual light reflexes, he responded to pain, and had semi-purposeful movements with the right arm only. There was no blood in his ears and nose. On examination he had a haematoma of the right parietal region and a scalp laceration of the left parietal region which was sutured in the casualty department. There was no movement in his left arm and limited movement in the left leg. In fact, his left side was quite weak and flaccid. He had an upgoing plantar reflex on the left side. He was catheterized in the casualty department.

A computerized tomography (CT) scan done through the casualty department revealed a right fronto-parietal haemorrhage with midline shift, so he was given dexamethasone and mannitol. He was also taken to the operating theatre and had a right burr hole and a brain needle aspiration for a clot. He was given phenytoin 250 mg intramuscularly on arrival and 25 mg intravenously, and dexamethasone 4 mg four times daily. After 2 days, his pupils were equal in size. His blood pressure was 160/90 mmHg, and he had a temperature of 38°C. He was seen to have had 2 to 3 episodes of fitting during that day. On discussion with the consultant he was placed on an antibiotic (cephalothin) and commenced on a diuretic (frusemide 40 mg) intravenously after having been given mannitol. His focal fitting continued so a brain needle was placed through the burr hole and a liquifying haemotoma type fluid was evacuated. His focal fitting settled. On the sixth day after injury his pupils became sluggish, and he was reacting to pain only. On review by the consultant, a further brain needle was placed through the burr hole and 10 ml of clot was removed. His pupilary reactions improved and he continued to make responses to pain. On the seventh day he opened his left eye spontaneously and the pupils were found to be equal and reacting. He was moving his right arm spontaneously. That day he had a repeat CT scan post contrast, which revealed that a clot was still present with now only a small amount of midline shift.

He continued to make little progress neurologically, but 17 days after the accident he began to show signs of recovery and began conversing appropriately with his mother. On the nineteenth day after brain injury, findings on neurological examination revealed a left hemianopia and a flaccid weakness on the left arm and leg. Intermittent words were spoken appropriately but conversation at that stage was not fluent. He was discharged to a rehabilitation hospital 37 days after the accident. Up to this stage he had made good improvement neurologically although he continued to have flaccid weakness on the left side. He had recovered speech but at times appeared to be confused and became disruptive to the staff with his constant calling out for assistance.

He was an inpatient at the rehabilitation hospital for treatment and vocational training for 15 months. He subsequently attended the neurological rehabilitation group for

CASE HISTORY — Male, aged 22 years cont.

physiotherapy for a year and a half and was also currently attending a college for work retraining in the field of computers The patient's main problem was left sided spasticity affecting his gait and giving him a non-functional left arm. He was walking without aid, but his gait faults were:

- During left swing phase: a rigid leg with no knee flexion or extension; all movement was coming from the pelvis rather than complementary pelvic/hip/knee movement; and a very long step forward.
- During left leg stance phase: poor weight shift to the left leading to short stance phase; poor weight shift forwards leading to a shortstep with the right leg; knee hyperextension.
- The patient had slight active shoulder movement but all movements resulted in an increase in tone causing his arm to internally rotate and his fingers to flex tightly.

Acupressure therapy began in January 1989 in Melbourne, (3 years and 10 months after the initial trauma). The clinical findings during his first visit for acupressure therapy, and the result of treatment are shown in Table 5.3.

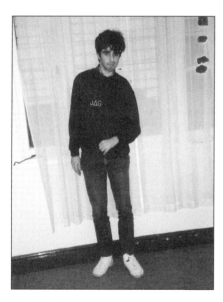

Fig. 5.1 Patient before treatment

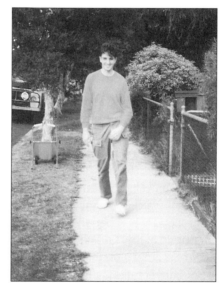

Fig. 5.2 Patient after treatment. He walks in the street

Table 5.3 Results of treatment

Before treatment	After treatment
1. Gait	
Walking with a limp and sluggish gait, left arm flexed and held close to the chest	The limp and sluggish gait improved. Left arm stretched with a little floxion in elbow joint, and with movement of left arm
Walking unstable	Walking more stable
Gait unsteady	Gait more stable
2. Left arm and hand	
Movement in left shoulder elbow and dropped wrist joints very limited	Movement in left shoulder and elbow joints normal but with a slight drop wrist
Flexion contracture of all fingers and thumb	Flexed contracture of thumb and fingers improved and some movement in little finger
Supination of forearm limited	Supination of forearm in normal range
Grasp power of left hand 4 kg	Grasp power of left hand 10 kg
3. Hip joint	
Stretch and elevation of left leg to 0°	Stretch and elevation of left leg actively 80°
Internal and external rotation limited	Internal and external rotation improved to near normal range
4. Left knee joint	
Left knee joint rigid, only a little flexion and extension	Left knee joint movement, both flexion and extension in normal range, but a little flaccid and unstable during swing phase
5. Left ankle joint and foot	
Drop foot	Corrected
Equinovarus	Corrected

CASE HISTORY— *Male, aged 22 years*

The patient's chief complaint was multiple functional handicaps after a car accident, 3 years and 6 months before his first visit in May 1989. Following the accident, the patient was unconscious for about 5 weeks and subsequently was in post traumatic amnesia for about 4 months. He was managed initially in an intensive care unit according to the referral information and required a tracheostomy and left sided intercostal drain tube because of pneumothorax. A fractured humerus was pinned 5 days after the accident, and a CT scan performed the following day showed diffuse cerebral oedema and petechial haemorrhages. The diagnosis was as follows:

A severe closed head injury
Fractured midshaft of left humerus
Fractured left scapula
Left sided pneumothorax
Disrupted left knee with injury to the medial ligament.

The patient was transferred to another hospital for a rehabilitation assessment and programme almost 4 months after the injury. He was non-ambulant, sitting in a high-backed wheelchair with a splint on his left knee. He was totally dependent in all activities of daily living and required full assistance for feeding. He was incontinent of urine.

Physically, he had poor head and neck control, and plantar flexion contractures in both feet with marked increase in muscle tone in all four limbs, worse on the left side. He was able to perform automatic movement with his right arm.

His ongoing memory and orientation were poor. He had left sided facial weakness and poor function in the left hand. He showed great difficulty in learning new material of a verbal nature. His memory for nonverbal visual material was equally poor, and he had significant attention problems. His medical report indicated that the range of movement in his right wrist and fingers had improved, and his control of voluntary movement on the right side was better. Little improvement had been recorded in his left arm. The range of movement in the lower limbs had increased with more flexion which allowed better sitting balance.

There were higher level language difficulties with abstract tasks and his verbal learning remained limited. His speech was impaired and showed mixed dysarthria with a predominant spastic component.

He was discharged from inpatient care almost a year after transfer to the rehabilitation hospital and was to continue attending for an outpatient rehabilitation programme aimed at further improving his gait, transfers, wheelchair mobility, communication skills and cognitive function. At the time of discharge he had no useful functional contraction in his left elbow. In his right upper limb he had reduced wrist extension which limited functional movement.

Before acupressure therapy, he was receiving outpatient rehabilitation consisting of physiotherapy, occupational therapy and speech pathology at a Melbourne hospital. It was felt at this post-injury stage that little further significant functional improvement would occur and that, as a result of his head injury, he would be left with severe physical and cognitive deficits.

- **Acupressure treatment**

The patient came to the clinic for a 30 minute treatment session 5 times a week. The treatment described below was given.

- **Management of speech problem**

1. Pressing the following points (5 to 6 times each in one treatment):

- Chuigen (MA point) (see Fig. 2.3).
- Dicang (S4) (see Fig. 2.1).
- Lianquan (Ren 23) (see Fig. 2.1).
- Yamen (DU 15) (see Fig. 2.2).
- Chengjiang (Ren 24) (see Fig. 2.1).
- Zengyin (Extra 11) (see Fig. 2.3).

2. Pinching the upper and lower lips round the mouth to stimulate the Orbicularis oris and Levator anguli oris muscles.

3. Massaging along the submandibular region to relax the spasm of muscles connected to the hyoid bone, and to stimulate hypoglossal and mylohyoid nerves.

4. Massaging using thumb and index finger on the hyoid bone (20 times).

5. Massaging along both sides of larynx using thumb and middle finger to stimulate the Thyrohyoid and Inferior constrictor muscle of the pharynx and also to stimulate the Laryngeal muscles to relax muscle spasm.

6. Massaging on root of the tongue. The doctor's left thumb and index finger pinch and pull so as to protrude the tongue: the right index finger should be covered with a rubber finger-cot or glove and put into the mouth to press on and massage the root of the tongue about 10 times. Then draw the tongue out of the mouth, directly forwards and to the right and to the left moving it about 10 times for each direction.

7. Speech exercises:

- Pronunciation: A, E, I, O, U
- Phoneticize (combine sounds into syllables):
  Ba, Be, Bo, Bu
  Da, De, Do, Du
  Fa, Fe, Fo, Fu
  G, H, J, K, L, M, N, P, R, S, T, V, X, Y, Z (A, E, I, O, U).
- Words:
  Baby, boy, back
  Class, clap, clam
  Day, dog, due
  Face, feet, food
- Sentences:
  Progress gradually from speaking simple to speaking more complicated sentences.

CASE REPORT — Male, aged 22 years cont.

The patient pronounced words indistinctly at the beginning of treatment and his articulation was difficult. After 53 sessions of manipulation, he enunciated his words clearly and easily, and he used about three to four words in a sentence.

• Management of the left shoulder joint

Adduction and internal rotation contractures presented in the patient's left shoulder. He could elevate his left arm only to 80°. He could not touch his right ear behind his head and his ability to rub his frontal region with the proximal portion of his forearm was limited. Also he could not touch his spine with his thumb. As has been described in Chapter 3, we combined the methods of examination and acupressure treatment (see Figs 3.3, 3.4, 3.5 and 3.6). In the early stages of treatment, spasticity and contracture were present and the patient experienced discomfort with movement.

The doctor gave percussion and massage to relieve pain and relax the muscle spasm, and after 53 sessions of manipulation, all movements at the patient's left shoulder were near normal range.

• Management of deformities of left wrist and hand: drop wrist

1. Pressing the following points:

• Yangchi (SJ 4). Location: on the transverse crease of the dorsum of the wrist, in the depression lateral to the tendon of the Extensor digitorum muscle (see Fig. 2.2). Press this area 5 to 6 times.

• Jihui (MA point). Location: on the radial side 2 cm below the transverse cubital crease at the prominence of the Extensor digitorum and Extensor carpi radialis longus muscles. Press this region 5 to 6 times for one treatment.

2. Percussion along the dorsal aspect of wrist and hand, and on the posterior aspect of forearm to increase the muscle tone.

3. Percussion and massage on the Flexor digitorum profundus and superficialis, Flexor carpi radialis and Flexor carpi ulnaris muscles to relieve spasm and contracture of these muscles.

4. After the manipulations mentioned above the splint can be used.

• Correction of clawfingers and adduction deformity of the thumb

1. Percussion along the left forearm, wrist, fingers and thumb.

2. Pressing the following points:

• Yangchi (SJ 4) located as mentioned above.
• Yangxi (LI 5) Location: on the radial side of the wrist. When the thumb is extended and abducted, it is in the depression between the tendons of Extensor pollicis longus and Extensor pollicis brevis (see Fig. 2.3). This point is used to increase the abducting force and tilt the thumb. Press 5 to 6 times for one treatment.

3. Percussion along the Extensor digitorum and Extensor pollicis longus to increase muscle tone.

4. Percussion and massage of Flexor pollicis longus, and Flexor digitorum profundus and superficialis to relax spasm of these muscles. Subsequently, extend the fingers and thumb.

5. Massage with two thumbs on the palm with the wrist in dorsal flexion (see Fig. 3.8). to relieve the spasm and contracture of the intrinsic muscles of the hand. Hyperextend the fingers and thumb at the same time.

6. After these manipulations, application of the splint on the arm and hand.

In general, the splint can be used before manipulation, but for this patient, whose left hand had severe deformities, the splint could be used only after some correction through manipulation. The patient's left hand had not only wrist-drop but also clawfingers and stiff flexed contracture in the four medial metacarpophalangeal joints. The left thumb had an adduction deformity. The main reason for using a splint after treatment (see Fig. 3.12) is to support the wrist, fingers and thumb in a corrected position and so avoid the return of wrist-drop, clawfingers and adducted thumb. Removal of the splint at home enables functional exercises of the wrist, fingers and thumb to be carried out after treatment.

• Management of hip problems

Clinical assessment of the patient's hip joints showed the following:

- Limitation of abduction. The frog test was positive, with spasticity and contracture of the Adductor muscles (longus, magnus, gracilis and brevis) and the Pectineus muscle. It occured on both sides (see Fig. 3.16).
- Spasticity in internal and external rotation led to limitation of movement at the left and right hip joints, and any attempt to produce movements at the joints caused pain (see Figs 3.17 and 3.18).
- Flexion at the hip joints. On the right side flexion to 90°, and on the left side flexion to 45° was possible. This meant that the left side was abnormal due to spasticity of the Hamstring muscles which led to limitation in stepping with the left leg (see Fig. 3.19).
- Contracture of Rectus femoris and Tensor fasciae latae, Psoas major and Iliacus muscles. Clinical examination showed 4-form test positive on the left side. It led to difficulty in extension of the left hip joint in which turn led to flexion of the lumbar spine.

The manipulative treatment is the same as shown in Figures 3.20 and 3.21.

• Management of deformities in ankles and feet

As mentioned in Chapter 3, equinovarus deformity is the most common problem in brain damaged patients and also in patients with cerebral birth injury and strokes. In the case of this patient, equinovarus was present on both sides which made standing and walking difficult. The manipulations for correction of equinovarus are as described over the page.

CASE REPORT — *Male, aged 22 years cont.*

1. Percussion and massage along the Tibialis anterior muscle.

2. With the patient in the prone position, pressing on the sole and percussion and massage along the Gastrocnemius muscle for correction of equine deformity.

3. With the patient in the supine position and the knee joint extended, pushing on the sole and dorsiflexion of the foot.

4. As shown in Figure 3.45, correction of drop foot by compression over the knee. This is repreated 30 times in one treatment.

5. By pulling the forefoot, correction of the inversion deformity at the tarsal joints (see Fig. 3.47).

6. Splints for external fixation, the plastic splint can be used. The fixation includes the ankle joint in dorsal flexion and the knee joint extended. It can be taken off at home during manipulation, but is used until the deformity is corrected (see Fig. 3.23).

• **Results of treatment**

The results after 53 treatments of acupressure therapy over 2 months are outlined in Table 5.4.

The following is a comment on the acupressure therapy from the patient:

The acupressure therapy has worked wonders in both my physical state and my mental attitude. In all, I'd personally like to thank Professor for opening doors to me that I thought were locked. For giving me another chance. For making pain enjoyable.

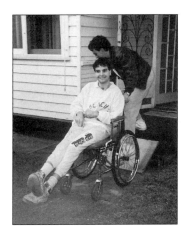

Fig. 5.3 Patient before treatment

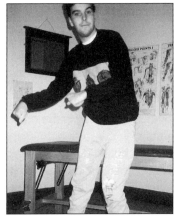

Fig. 5.4 Patient after treatment

Table 5.4 Results of treatment

Before treatment	After treatment
1. Mental condition Amnesia, on-going memory poor. Concentration lost after less than half an hour. Difficulty in dealing with abstract verbal concepts, difficulty in solving arithmetical problems, very poor capacity to analyze a problem, plan a solution, carry out a task, and recognize and correct errors made	Reduced irritability. Memory improved and also the ability to plan in advance; increased positivity and efficiency
2. Speech Speech impaired with a mixed dysarthria and a predominate spastic component. Speech slow, slurred, with rigidity of the tongue. Difficulty in talking with others	In the patient's own words, 'This is the greatest, and most obvious improvement'. Speech much louder, much faster and more coherent
3. Head and neck control poor	Head and neck control good
4. Left shoulder elevation to 80°. Unable to touch opposite ear	Left shoulder elevation to 130° much improved. Patient feels the arm is looser
Unable to touch spine	Improved
5. Supination of left forearm limited	Some degree of improvement
6. Abduction contracture of left thumb, limited movement	Improved. Range of movement near normal
7. Clawfingers, flexion contracture of metacarpophalangeal joints	Improved
8. Grasp (2 May 89), left hand 0 kg, right hand 18 kg	Grasp (11 July 89), left hand 0.3 kg, right hand 15 kg
9. Able to stand with support of two hands for about 2 minutes	Able to stand with support of one hand for more than 10 minutes
10. Able to walk with the help of two people; limped in left leg, and had difficulty in making a step; equinovarus and inner rotation of left foot present	Walks with the help of one person; limp and equinovarus much improved and walks faster and more easily

Table 5.4 Results of treatment cont.

Before treatment	After treatment
11. Hip joints Abduction limited	Abduction of hip joints near normal
Both internal and external rotation limited	Both internal and external rotation in normal range
Stretch and elevation of legs: right side 90° (normal); left side 45° (abnormal)	Right side 90°; left side 89° (near normal range)
12. Equinovarus present on both sides, minimal on right side	Completely corrected on right side, and improved on left side

CHAPTER 6

CEREBROVASCULAR ACCIDENTS

A cerebrovascular accident (CVA) or 'stroke' is defined as the clinical expression of a pathologic process involving the cerebral vasculature, either directly or indirectly, and resulting in a secondary abnormality of the brain (Sutin 1986). Cerebrovascular accidents are one of the most common causes of morbidity and mortality in the world. A stroke can be produced by a variety of conditions involving the intracranial and extracranial vessels as well as some systemic diseases. The primary symptoms vary according to the neural tissues damaged by the cerebrovascular accident. The secondary problems that patients suffer are often either consequences of, or complications following, the primary lesion.

VASCULAR DISORDERS AFFECTING THE BRAIN

Obstructive vascular disease may be considered as a continuum, extending from mild, 'transient', isolated or repetitive manifestations to ultimate, maximal and permanent neurologic deficit. The clinical types are described in the next pages.

Haemorrhagic stroke

Hypertension is the most frequent cause of intracerebral haemorrhage. The other common predisposing factors include haemorrhagic diathesis, liver disease, anticoagulation, brain tumours, mycotic aneurysms and haemophilia. Haemorrhagic stroke occurs without prodromal stage or warning and in middle aged people with poorly controlled blood pressure. The patient is usually awake and active at onset.

Clinical manifestations are as follows:

- Headache is a common symptom in about half the stroke patients. Other symptoms include nausea and vomiting. Bleeding closer to the surface of the brain is more likely to result in headache.
- Neck rigidity occurs as a result of blood entering the subarachnoid space. Examination of cerebrospinal fluid shows the presence of red cells.
- Vomiting is a frequent occurrence in cerebral haemorrhage, regardless of the site involved. It is associated with a lesion in the anterior circulation typically attributable to haemorrhage.
- Hemiplegia.
- Unconsciousness.
- Bleeding in the dominant temporal area produces asphasia, homonymous hemianopia, memory deficits, apraxia, or visual problems.
- Bleeding in the medial frontal region produces abulia, incontinence and prominent or suck reflexes.
- Large posterior haemorrhages result in brain stem compression and displacement, such as putamenal haemorrhage penetrating to the sub-arachnoid space.

- The size of the haemorrhage mass may vary from 1-3 cm, which is small, to 7-8 cm, which is likely to be fatal. In determining the size and the site of haemorrhagic mass by the use of computerized transaxial tomography flow (CT) or magnetic resonance imaging (MRI), the extended capacity of visualization by CT or MRI scans enables small differences in the densities of the various tissues of the brain and the surrounding structures to be identified.

- Symptoms of cerebellar haemorrhage arise with surprising suddenness, and the entire course is often extremely brief: stupor followed by coma, and death within 48 hours. Localizing symptoms of cerebellar haemorrhage include cranial nerve palsies, headache, nausea, vomiting, inability to walk, dizziness, mild ipsilateral peripheral facial weakness, ipsilateral decreased corneal response, ipsilateral sixth nerve palsy, oscillopsia, unilateral or bilateral internuclear ophthalmoplegia, nystagmus, paresis or lateral gaze to the side of haemorrhage, or forced conjugate gaze to the opposite side, loss of balance, limb ataxia, no sensory loss, no hemiplegia, and pyramidal signs. The occurrence of respiratory failure may be due to secondary pressure on the pontine and medullary areas.

- Thalamic haemorrhage. This is characterized by the onset of sensory loss which precedes motor loss and tends to be more prominent. The motor deficits occur as a result of pressure on the adjacent internal capsule after a latent period. Multiple deficits of high brain stem origin are seen. If the nuclei of the upper midbrain are involved, eye problems result.

- Haemorrhage of the pons results in coma within several minutes with rapid respiration, headache, vomiting, quadriparesis, pinpoint reactive pupils, and other problems of the eyes.

- Haemorrhage of the brain stem, where the clinical symptoms are very severe, may cause coma and death.
- Brain haemorrhage due to rupture of a cerebral aneurysm is a frequent cause of subarachnoid haemorrhage, and often occurs during physical exertion. The clinical signs are sudden intense headache, stupor without paralysis, nausea, vomiting, stiff neck, and oculomotor palsy. The age of the typical patient is early fifties for both sexes. The CSF shows large amounts of blood; neck pain and pain on eye movement and refractory vomiting are common.

Embolic strokes

The onset of embolic events is swift, with no warning. Usually the deficit occurs within seconds or minutes and a secondary deficit follows. The onset is most often during waking hours, or it can occur just as the patient steps out of bed. Embolic material most often consists of fibrin-platelet aggregates, atherosclerotic debris, or cholesterol plaques. Clinically, embolism is often seen in the younger patient. Regarding clinical onset, embolic strokes can be characterized as painless, with relatively clear consciousness; often epileptic seizures are associated with embolism. Cardiac dysrhythmias are present in the majority of patients with cerebral embolism, and postmyocardial infarction or prosthetic valve replacement are also a significant precipitating cause (Sutin 1986).

Cerebral emboli have been documented in association with multiple cardiac pathological changes, for example, rheumatic heart disease with mitral stenosis and atrial fibrillation.

Thrombotic strokes

The onset of a thrombotic stroke may be sudden, but it tends to evolve more slowly and is often preceded by transient ischaemic attacks. Patients are usually in their early sixties, and are frequently hypertensive or have cerebral atherosclerotic disease. It is also found in patients occluded with peripheral or coronary blood vessels, diabetes mellitus, gout, polycythaemia, xanthomatosis. The formation of a thrombus depends on a number of interrelated factors: local injury or roughening of the vascular wall, the viscosity and atrocrit of the blood, the number of platelets and their activation, and the presence of serum coagulant and anticoagulant substances.

Clinically, the onset occurs during sleep or continues to progress upon awakening. There is usually no pain and the patient remains conscious. Sometimes headache occurs, and bowel and bladder dysfunction and oedema. The gradualness of a slowly developing haemorrhage means it may present as a progressive thrombotic infarction. Motor recovery is very slow. Complications of heart disease are a common cause of death.

Transient ischaemic attacks

A transient ischaemic attack is an event characterized by focal neurologic deficit, from which the patient fully recovers within a 24 hour period.

Atherosclerosis of the major neck arteries (carotid and vertebral arteries) is the major cause of transient ischaemic attacks and leads to the onset of embolic and thrombotic strokes. Transient symptoms of cerebral ischaemia are frequently due to emboli which break off from ulcerated plaques and are carried to the brain. The resulting symptoms depend on the point at which the emboli obstruct the cerebral circulation and their onset is characteristically sudden, for example, blindness, numbness, weakness, clumsiness, paralysis of any combination of limbs up to quadriplegia, and paraesthesia or loss of sensation of varying extent. Headaches may accompany transient ischaemic attack, but are usually brief and not severe.

Factors increasing the deficit are as follows:

- Extension of the clot
- Embolization of a fresh, loosely adherent clot to a distal location, rendering that region more ischaemic
- Activation of platelets and other clotting factors that enhance coagulability
- Vulnerability of the particular brain tissue to hypoxia and hypoperfusion.

Other factors that act to decrease the deficit are as follows:

- Rapid development of collateral circulation
- Activation of fibrinolytic and thrombolitic mechanisms which tend to lyse the clot
- Adherence of the clot to the vessel wall which makes it less likely that embolism will occur later
- Fragmentation of emboli which pass through the vascular bed, thus opening previously blocked branches
- Resistance of some tissues to hypoxia and hypoperfusion. Such tissues remain tenuous for the first days or weeks.

The clinical task is to promote natural factors that are working toward minimizing the deficit.

Thus, the treatment should be aimed at the clinical ischaemic problems, the low blood flow and blood clotting with embolization within the vessels; treatment should also be directed towards improving the resistance of the brain to ischaemia, bringing more blood to the area, or helping the brain to use the blood in the most effective way.

CARE OF THE ACUTE PATIENT

General treatment applies to all stroke patients. These general measures are described below.

- The maintenance of an effective airway and the institution of monitoring of responsiveness, especially in patients who are unconscious.
- The maintenance of blood pressure.
- As early as possible, determine the primary cause of the stroke and whether or not there is a need for an emergency operation for a patient who may have either a haemorrhage in the brain or a subdural haematoma.
- Bladder care. Initially, in-dwelling catheters are useful in preventing bladder overdistension; subsequently, intermittent catheterization with a straight catheter is useful in assisting the patient to re-establish normal bladder function.
- Skin care. Pressure ulcers may be avoided by frequent position changes, (the patient should have a position change every 2 hours for reduction of skin irritation), and the use of air, water flotation, sponge mattress or sheep skin, and massage with 50% alcohol aplied to vulnerable areas of the skin.
- Passive range of motion (ROM) exercises. Even before formal physiotherapy is initiated, nursing staff may begin ranging exercises on the paralyzed limbs to prevent contractures of joints.
- Early physiotherapy.

- Regulation of fluid and electrolyte balance: under normal conditions daily fluid intake should equal fluid loss. In the first 3-4 days after CVA when the patient finds eating and drinking difficult, fluid may need to be given intravenously in a glucose/saline combination. For an adult, an intake of between 1500 to 2000 ml per 24 hours may be necessary. The fluid balance would be monitored carefully.
- Nutrition of CVA patients: the total energy requirements, as in patients with brain injury, may be little different from normal. When starting nasogastric feeding one method is to use a combination of milk and water, 30-100 ml every hour. It is sufficient to supply 2000 to 3000 calories per day.
- Treatment of the underlying disease which caused the stroke should be ongoing at the same time. Treatment must be tailored to the individual patient and his or her particular problem.

Treatment of special conditions

Measures required may include the following:

- Surgical removal of the occluding lesion may be required.
- Endarterectomy may be required to open a vessel for relieving a vascular obstruction.
- Hypovolaemia and dehydration should be gradually corrected and congestive heart failure should be treated.
- For increasing blood flow to a specific area, vasodilating agents may be considered.
- Heparin, warfarin, and antiplatelet agglutinating agents (for example, indomethecin, phenylbutazone and aspirin) may be used for their regulating anticoagulant effect.

ACUPRESSURE THERAPY

Contraindications

The use of acupressure therapy is contraindicated in CVA patients under the following conditions:

1. In the acute stage of cerebrovascular accident and for 6 months after a stroke attack. For paralyzed patients, early passive movements of limbs, especially the joint movements, are necessary. It is important to prevent deformities of the extremities.

2. Haemorrhagic diseases such as haemophilia, haemorrhagic purpura, allergic purpura, thrombopenic purpura, and patients with abnormal bleeding and coagulation time.

3. Severe heart diseases.

4. Tuberculosis, malignant tumours, and the acute stage of pyogenic arthritis.

5. Severe skin diseases.

6. Hypertension, where the blood pressure is higher than 160/100 mmHg.

When some patients with hypertension suffer a CVA, the blood pressure is reduced to a normal level. Under these conditions there is no contraindication for acupressure therapy.

Points for attention

The following points require attention in clinical practice:

1. When an anticoagulant is taken there is a tendency to haemorrhage.

2. Determination of blood pressure, pulse rate, bleeding and coagulation time, and pulmonary and urinary bladder conditions are very important, especially in elderly patients.

3. If the patient suffers a fall, the curative effect can regress, and treatment may need to be stopped until the patient recovers, particularly in cases of fracture such as a femur neck fracture in the elderly.

4. Do not neglect to ensure that the treatment of the primary disease such as heart disease, hypertension, and thromboangiitis is continuing while acupressure therapy is provided.

5. It is necessary to appreciate the many differences between patients who suffer cerebral birth injury, brain injury, and patients with cerebrovascular accident. The latter group is more complex and difficult to treat.

• The unconscious patient

Acupressure therapy can be done when the patient is unconscious. If the patient has suffered a CVA, he will be able to receive acupressure therapy, even though he is unconscious, after 6 months, and when none of the abovementioned six conditions of contraindication are present. The doctor may try pressing a few points for recovery of consciousness, such as:

- Yongquan (K1). Location: on the sole of the foot, in the depression when the foot is in plantar flexion, approximately at the junction of the anterior third and posterior two thirds of the sole (see Fig. 2.3).
- Bige (MA point). Location: there are 3 points around the root of nasal pillar (see Fig. 2.1).
- Zhijiagen (MA point) (see Fig. 2.2).

• Approach to treatment

The general approach to manipulation for patients with CVA should be noted. In the beginning the manipulation should be done gently, with mild stimulation, carefully weighing up the patient's words and closely watching his expression, and gradually increasing the strength of the manipulation. Tell the patient in advance that he will probably experience such sensations as soreness, numbness, warmth and distention in the area of manipulation. Skin flush may also occur, and subcutaneous small bleeding may occur at the beginning of treatment. It will usually disappear within one week.

There are some obvious limitations in shoulder and hip joints. It is not necessary for these to be corrected to the extent recommended for children, who are more likely to reach the normal range of movement. Repeat the manipulations carefully and always stop before going too far. On the other hand, the goal of minimal functional requirement should be achieved, such as holding objects, palms touching face, sitting, standing and even walking.

• Frequency of treatment

The treatment for adult patients should be carried out either every day, 5 sessions in a week, or every other day, or twice weekly, according to the condition of the individual patient. Usually 60 sessions over 3 months constitute one course of treatment, because the curative effect tends to decrease after 3 months. The second course may start after 4-6 weeks' interval, when there will be new progress.

For children who are CVA patients, the treatment may be given once every day. The first course may finish within 3 months. The second course is the same as mentioned above for adults.

Visual dysfunction

Visual disturbances such as anopia, hemianopia, and optic atrophy are common in stroke patients. The method of treatment is the same as the technique used in treating visual problems in patients with cerebral birth injury (see Ch. 3).

Communication disorders

Many patients experience speech problems after a stroke, including aphasia, dysphasia and aphonia. The application of Chinese acupressure therapy is effective in adult stroke cases of dysphasia and aphasia. However, in children with dysphasia and aphasia associated with cerebral birth injury, the gains are very limited.

• **Manipulations for speech**

1. Pressing the following points 5 to 6 times in one treatment with the tip of the finger:

• Chuigen (MA point). Location: just below the earlobe, both sides (see Fig. 3.66).
• Chengjiang (Ren 24). Location: in the depression in the centre of the mentolabial groove (see Fig. 3.68).
• Lianquan (Ren 23). Location: above the prominence of the larynx, in the depression at the level of the upper border of the hyoid bone (see Fig. 3.68).
• Yamen (DU 15). Location: 1.5 cm directly above the mid point of the posterior hairline, in the depression below the spinous process of the first cervical vertebra (see Fig. 2.2).
• Yifeng (SJ 17). Location: posterior to the lobe of the ear, in the depression between the mandible and mastoid process (see Fig. 2.2).

2. Massage along the submandibular region (see Fig. 3.71) to relax and reduce contracture of the underlying tongue muscles and muscles stabilizing the hyoid bone. This procedure is aimed at increasing the mobility of the hyoid bone, to promote the movement of the tongue and hence to improve speech. Then, with the thumb and index finger touching both sides of the hyoid bone massage forwards and backwards along the bone. Repeat both procedures about 20 times in one treatment. This, and other treatments described below should be carried out once daily.

3. Massaging the root of the tongue. Ask the patient to open the mouth as wide as possible, and then to put out the tongue. With a gauze pad in left hand, the doctor pulls the tongue out further. The gloved index finger of the other hand is used to press and massage the root of the tongue. Repeat about 10 times in one treatment. After this, two hands are used to hold the anterior part of the tongue and pull outwards to the right side, to the left side and straight ahead with gentle movements about 10 times in one treatment (each side).

4. Massaging up and down along both sides of the laryngopharynx about 20 times.

5. Pressing point Zengyin (Extra 11). Location: 3 cm behind and at the level of the prominence of the larynx. Press 5 to 6 times in one treatment.

In CVA patients the speech problem may be due to cortical damage, or to secondary factors which cause muscle spasm or stiffness. The absence of natural tone in the muscles causes clinical manifestation in speech problems.

Shoulder joint problems

The shoulder is the site of a number of complications after CVA. Clinical manifestations often include tendonitis, bursitis, adhesive capsulitis, rotator cuff tear, glenohumeral subluxation, shoulder-hand syndrome, and fracture of the humeral surgical neck. The shoulder-hand syndrome is a clinical entity involving pain, oedema, and loss of motion in the upper extremity.

Clinical manifestations are pain over the shoulder joint. There are 8 painful points as follows (see Figs 6.1 and 6.2):

1. Anteriorly, the site of the tendon sheath of the long head of Biceps muscle

2. Posteriorly, the origin of the head of Triceps muscle

3. Laterally, the midpoint of the origin of Deltoid muscle

4. The origin of Supraspinatus

5. The centre of Infraspinatus

6. The upper angle of the scapula

7. The midpoint of spinal border of the scapula

8. The lower angle of the scapula.

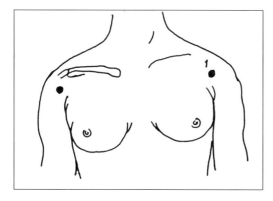

Fig. 6.1 Painful points around the shoulder joint. Anterior view

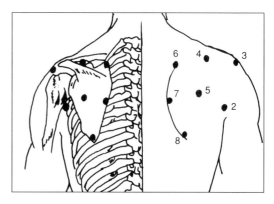

Fig. 6.2 Painful points around the shoulder joint. Posterior view

Other clinical manifestations include stiffness of the shoulder joint, limitation of movement, and functional disturbance in the arm.

• **Manipulation for shoulder joint**

1. Press on and massage the painful point; general percussion around the shoulder.

2. Four functional movements should be done. These are described in Chapter 3, which should be referred to. Doctors should note the difference in treatment for children and adults. For the elderly it is not necessary to reach the full range of movement for all manipulations.

3. In the treatment for glenohumeral subluxation, we often use a shoulder-elbow plaster splint, together with manipulation of the shoulder. The splint can be taken off and reapplied after each treatment.

• **Management of shoulder-hand problems**
Apply mild percussion over the whole arm; find the painful points and press them 5 to 6 times for one treatment; put a hot compress on each of the affected areas for 20 minutes for one treatment every day.

Chinese herbs in the form of a decoction were given in some cases to promote blood circulation, decrease oedema and relieve pain. With this treatment, the clinical symptoms indicated that recovery was very fast, usually after 3-4 weeks. (The total treatment included pressing painful points, percussion generally, and hot compresses, as well as the herb decoction.)

Difficulties in stretching a spastic arm

When working with patients with spastic contracture of shoulder, elbow, wrist and even fingers, it is important that the doctors or other therapists do not use force to obtain the stretch. This only meets with difficulty or defeat in practice. In our experience, it is more successful to start manipulation with gentle percussion on the whole arm, along the six stimulation lines, for 4-5 minutes. At the same time, the doctor's other hand gently facilitates passive movements in the joints.

1. After general percussion, the treatment may go on to the following 'trigger' points which we have found useful in our practice. These are located as follows:

   a. Biceps. On Biceps muscle located in the lower third of the muscle. Press it with thumb and give some upward, downward movement along the muscle for 4-5 minutes. At the same time as the patient's arm is stretched, it becomes easier to extend.

   b. Brachioradialis. On Brachioradialis muscle, at the antero-lateral of the elbow joint. Press it with the thumb on the upper part of this muscle. The other operating procedures are the same as above.

   c. Superficial flexor. At the origin of the superficial Flexors of the forearm located on the antero-medial aspect of the elbow joint. Press on the upper part of these muscles near their origins. The technique is as above.

2. Press point Yangchi (SJ 4). Location: on the transverse crease of the dorsum of the wrist, in the depression lateral to the tendon of the Extensor digitorum muscle (see Fig. 2.2). Use the tip of the thumb, index or middle finger for percussion, 5 to 6 times to relax the flexion contracture of fingers.

3. Press point Yangxi (L15). Location: on the radial side of the wrist. When the thumb is

tilted upward, it is found in the 'anatomical snuff-box', the depression between the tendons of Extensors pollicis longus and brevis (see Fig. 2.3). The manipulative technique is the same for pressing point Yangchi (SJ 4). The purpose is to relax the flexion contracture of the thumb.

4. After pressing these points, the treatment may move on to massage along the spastic muscle or muscle groups. It is performed by three finger massage, using the index, middle, and ring fingers. The tips of these fingers touch the affected muscle, gently moving and vibrating in order to relieve the spasm (contracture) of the muscle fibres. With three finger massage, work from the upper portion or origin of the muscle down to its insertion, 5 to 10 times in one treatment.

Forearm pronation deformity

Changes in tone and motor control of muscles often result in changes and imbalances of muscle groups around the joint; these changes and imbalances can result in deformities. The natural resting or sleeping position of the forearm is in pronation. After a stroke, brain injury or cerebral birth injury many patients have complications with pronation contracture of the forearm resulting in the limitation of supination of the forearm. This leads to severe dysfunction in the upper limb.

Anatomically, the forearm pronation deformity is due to contracture or spasm of the pronator muscles such as Brachioradialis, Pronator teres, and Pronator quadratus muscles. It may also be due to weakness of the supinator muscles such as Supinator and Biceps muscles. The manipulations for correction of forearm pronation deformity are the same as in patients with cerebral birth injury, or brain damage due to injury later (see Fig. 3.7).

External fixation by the use of a splint (plaster or plastic) may be used to support and maintain the forearm in the supination position. It is applied during patient treatment in the out-patient department (after manipulation), and is also for use at home when the clinical course is finished. The splint is often used in cases where deformity cannot be corrected by manipulation alone. The plaster case should be maintained for 3-4 weeks. The plaster should extend from the middle portion of the upper arm to the tips of the fingers with the forearm fully extended.

Deformities of the wrist and hand

Motor and sensory deficits, spasticity, and joint contractures cause very obvious deformities of the wrist, thumb and fingers. Marked spasticity in the wrist and finger and thumb flexors in palmar flexion lead to deformity of the wrist, fixed fingers, or clenched fists with the thumb in the palm. The patient is unable to open his fingers.

• **Correction of drop wrist**

Through percussion along the forearm, over the wrist and fingers, and by stretching fingers and wrist, it is possible to relax the muscles in a short time. Massage along the Flexor carpi radialis and Flexor carpi ulnaris, Flexor digitorum superficialis, Flexor digitorum profundus, and Flexor pollicis longus muscles to release the flexion contracture in the fingers and thumb. Massage on the thenar area to release adduction contracture of the thumb.

There are two reasons for applying hand splints (see Figs 3.10 and 3.12):

- To support the wrist and fingers in a straight position just after manipulation
- To enable fixation and functional exercises.

The effect of acupressure therapy locally on the area being treated, is to decrease the high tone of spastic muscles. Experience has provided conclusive evidence for me that acupressure manipulation can relax spastic muscles. It is, as a result, an appreciated and, for me, the preferred method of treatment. The functional exercises are the same as described in Chapter 3. Surgical management is indicated in some cases, but this is not the place to give details. However, I wish to stress the effectiveness of acupressure therapy in postoperative treatment.

Hip deformities after stroke

In the early stages of recovery following a cerebro-vascular accident, physiotherapy manipulation may be administered in the patient's hospital room and bed in order to prevent muscle tightness and contractures, maintain skin integrity, inhibit abnormal posture and muscle tone, and stimulate muscle activity and function. Even though the therapists achieve great success in their work, it is still clear that such manipulation frequently does not prevent the development of severe complications in the upper and lower limbs. In order to determine the functional disturbance in the hip joint, the tests described below are used in the initial clinical examination.

Frog test
This tests the extent of abduction at the hip joint for adduction contracture of the hip and posterior dislocation of the hip joint.

Internal rotation of the hip joint

This test is to determine the presence of spasm or contracture of the external rotator muscles of the hip joint.

Stretch and elevation of leg

This test is to determine contracture or weakness of the Biceps femoris, Semimembranosus, Semitendinosus posteriorly, and Rectus femoris, Tensor fasciae latae muscles, and the Flexors of the thigh anteriorly.

The 4-form test in prone position (see Fig. 3.22)

This test is for observation of spasm or contracture of the Rectus femoris, Iliopsoas and the fascia lata). A patient who is found to be positive in the 4-form test, stands or walks with flexion in the lumbar region and finds extension of the trunk difficult; big steps are limited during walking and there is difficulty with extension at the hip joint.

Ober's test (sign)

This test is to determine contracture of iliotibial tract. Ober's sign is often positive in patients who suffer cerebral birth injury, brain damage or cerebrovascular accident (stroke). Sometimes one side is affected and sometimes both. The patient with iliotibial tract contracture walks on a wide base with a stiff legged gait or sway steps.

After examination, the therapists go on to summarize the positive findings, and work out a programme for treatment. The technique of examination is combined with treatment. For example, in the correction of adduction deformity of the hip joint, the practitioner may put the legs in the frog position, so that the thighs are abducted at the hip joints; at the same time the adductor muscles of the thigh, which are likely to be in spasm, are stretched and become painful.

What more can be done at this moment? Does the therapist stop or go on? The answer is not to give way to impatience. The therapist keeps his forearms on the patient's flexed knee joints, and puts one of his hands on the upper part of each of the patient's thighs with the thumbs and thenar eminence on the tight spastic adductor muscle groups. As massage to relieve the spasm continues, some progress may be felt in the extension of the hip joints. If this manipulation is repeated about 40 to 50 times every day, the adductor contractures of the hip joint may be corrected and a normal range of movement achieved. The procedure described above is suitable for children, and young people under 30. For people in the 40-60 age group or more, the manipulations for correction of deformities in hip joints or other places should be treated carefully. I wish to stress once more the importance of careful manipulation, to ensure that you stop before going too far. This is necessary to prevent fractures and any damage.

After manipulation has been used to expand hip abduction to nearer the normal range, the frog splint is applied to hold this range for as long as possible, until the patient cannot bear it any longer. The longer the fixation the better, day time or night time, until the adductor contracture is completely corrected.

Manipulation for internal and external rotation at the hip joint may be carried out with the lower limb straight or flexed at the knee joint. In elderly patients care must be taken to avoid fracture of the neck of the femur, but a total range of 50° - 60° of rotation may be achieved at the hip joint over a period of time. When you find muscle spasm or resistance, give percussion directly along those muscles, which is very effective for relieving the muscular contractures. For children and young people under 30 the manipulation should reach 90° (normal range).

Iliotibial tract contracture

This deformity is rarely seen in CVA patients. The method of treatment is the same as for cerebral birth injury (see Figs 3.20 and 3.21). For the elderly, manipulation involves only percussion and massage along the iliotibial tract of the affected thigh with a mild adduction motion with the knee joint in a flexed position.

Treatment to relieve contracture of the Rectus femoris, Sartorius, and Iliopsoas is by the use of 4-form position with the patient in the prone position (see Fig. 3.22). Put one hand on the gluteal region and push down. The other hand holds the knee joint flexed at 90°; push the knee inward and upward. Repeat 20 times in one treatment. Massage along the Rectus femoris to relieve the contracture of this muscle from its origin to its insertion; repeat about 20-30 times. Press on a point which is located 3 cm lateral to the anterior superior iliac spine; one can feel the knee become relaxed. Also press another point, of benefit to relax the contracture preventing normal flexion of the knee: Heding (Extra 31). This is located in the depression at the midpoint of the superior border of the patella.

It is sometimes necessary to address the problem of how to maintain the knee joint in an extended position? In one patient who suffered haemorrhagic stroke with quadriplegia for 10 months, before treatment the knee joints were flexed to 60°. After 2 months manipulative treatment both knees could be extended to 150° although it was difficult to maintain the knee joints in this position for any length of time. We therefore began a programme of continuous traction. After manipulation, applied at the level of the ankle joints, a thick sponge (5 cm) was placed around the joints, under traction belts attached to a weight of 4 to 5 kilograms. (This is the traction weight suitable for adults, but for children, the weight should be according to the age). The traction on this patient was maintained until the deformity was corrected.

The other problem associated with knee flexion contracture is fibrous adhesion to the joint capsule. This means the patella cannot move, which greatly inhibits ready correction of the contracture. When we found fibrous adhesion in our clinical practice, we developed a manipulative treatment to overcome the problem. Two movements were used at the beginning of each treatment session: pushing the patella upwards and downwards, and massaging around the patella.

This procedure greatly facilitated the subsequent stretching of the flexion contracture of the knee joint.

Knee flexion contracture and drop foot

Another important aspect of knee flexion contracture became apparent during our clinical practice. The condition was usually associated with the presence of drop foot, especially in children and young patients. This combination of knee flexion contracture and drop foot was rarely found in elderly patients.

The following is a description of this combination and its treatment in a young boy who attended our clinic. This patient had suffered am embolic stroke after a heart operation. He had quadriplegia with a flexion contracture in both knee joints. Correction of this deformity subsequently caused the occurrence of drop foot. Correction of the drop foot caused a relapse of knee flexion contracture. What was the reason for this condition and what could we do in further treatment?

Our understanding is that the knee flexion contracture may be the result of weakness of the

Quadriceps and Tensor fasciae latae muscles leading to reduced capacity to extend the knee joint and of contracture of the Hamstring and Gastrocnemius muscles. In stroke patients, knee flexion contracture is due to spasm of the Flexor muscles of the knee joint. The condition we describe as drop foot (that is plantar flexion at the ankle joint) is caused by unrestricted action of the Gastrocnemius muscles. Treatment of footdrop involves stretching the Gastrocnemius muscles by extending the knee joint while dorsiflexing the ankle joint.

In our experience, correction of drop foot and knee joint contracture should take place together. Treatment of one, without treatment of the other, only increases the problem in the other. Our treatment involves manipulation and external fixation (splinting) of both problem areas. This has proved to be a successful method of correcting the two deformities.

Some patients exhibit only drop foot with no appearance of flexion contracture of the knee joint. This gives the wrong impression that there is only one problem to be corrected. When the drop foot is corrected, this causes the appearance of flexion contracture at the knee joint.

Where patients exhibit flexion contracture at the knee joint with no appearance of drop foot, once again there is a false impression of a single problem area. Correction of one causes deformity in the other. Treatment involves acupressure therapy and manipulative techniques, combined with splinting to maintain extension at the knee joint and dorsiflexion at the ankle joint. This has proved highly successful. In some cases, where surgical treatment is still found to be necessary, acupressure therapy and manipulation has assisted the recuperation of the patient.

Knee extension deformity

This deformity is the common disability seen in stroke patients due to extensor synergy, the effect of gravity, and a variable degree of tone in the Quadriceps muscle, during terminal stance and initial swing phase of walking, preventing knee flexion and causing a stiff-legged gait.

Management for the above described condition is as follows:

1. Give percussion along the anterior aspect of the thigh for about 5 minutes.

2. Hold the Quadriceps and move it medially and laterally.

3. Flex the knee joint.

4. Massage around the patella over the joint space 20 to 30 times in one treatment.

Surgical release of the Vastus intermedius and Rectus femoris has resulted in improved ambulation, but we suggest that it be performed only after manipulative treatment.

Knee extension deformity may also be the result of weakness of the Hamstring muscles. The management is as follows:

1. Percussion is applied to the Hamstrings for 5 to 10 minutes.

2. Percussion of the Gastrocnemius muscle 5 to 10 minutes.

3. If external fixation is needed, flexion of the knee joint to 160° should be maintained for 4 to 5 hours a day and even at night, until the deformity is corrected.

Ankle and foot

My personal experience and observation of ankle and foot problems is that patients with cerebrovascular accident, cerebral birth injury, and brain damage have similar conditions such as drop foot, heel foot, equinovarus, equinovalgus, inversion of the foot, eversion of the foot, clawtoes, and clawfoot. However there are some differences in the incidence of these deformities.

Equinovarus is more often found in Chinese and Japanese patients, perhaps due to the Chinese custom of sitting with crossed legs rather than with the feet in an inverted position. The Japanese are used to the 'camel' position, sitting on inverted feet. These positions result in inversion or equinovarus deformities.

Everted foot or equinovalgus occurs more in Australian patients, perhaps due to the Australian children sitting more in a 'W' or 'M' form position, i.e., squatting with both knee joints flexed, the feet turned outward and the bottom put on the flexed legs and outward turning feet. The severity of the deformity seems worse in children.

Drop foot

This is a common deformity. The patient has a problem clearing the toes from the ground during the swing phase of walking and decreased basal support during stance phase. It may be the result of weakness in the Tibilalis anterior, Extensor digitorum longus, and Extensor hallucis longus muscles, and spasticity in the Gastrocnemius and Tibialis posterior muscles. The manipulative technique is as follows:

1. Percussion along the dorsiflexor muscles of the foot to increase muscle tone.

2. Percussion and three-finger massage along the Gastrocnemius muscle and the sole of the foot with the foot in dorsal flexion. The patient is in the prone position (see Fig. 3.46).

3. External fixation using a splint. The ankle joint is in dorsal flexion and the knee joint extended.

Equinovarus

This is also a common deformity in CVA patients. The Tibialis anterior muscle and not the Posterior tibialis muscle is the culprit. The manipulative technique is as follows:

1. Percussion and massage along Tibialis anterior is required to relax the spasm.

2. Manipulation of the foot (see Fig. 3.47).

3. Pushing the foot from the sole to a position of dorsal flexion with the knee joint extended.

4. External fixation with the knee extended and the foot in dorsal flexion, for 4 to 6 weeks. The splint can be taken off during manipulation. Surgical correction can be carried out if the deformity does not respond to manipulative treatment.

Equinovalgus

This is a more common deformity in CVA patients and also in cerebral birth injury and brain damage cases, due to spasm or contracture of the Peroneus longus and Peroneus brevis muscles. Treatment is as follows:

1. Percussion and massage along the Peroneal muscles.

2. Pushing the foot into a position of dorsal flexion and eversion. Repeat about 30 times.

3. External fixation as for equinovarus. Surgical treatment can be used after conservative therapy.

CASE HISTORY — *Male, aged 2 years 3 months*

Date of first visit 15 April 1989, date of onset of illness 17 April 1987. The patient suffered brain damage when he was 14 weeks old. He suffered congenital heart disease for which he was operated on at 14 weeks of age. After the operation his heart condition was very good, but 5 hours later he had a heart arrest and suffered brain damage. He was also cortically blind. The brain CT scan shows diffused infarct lesions in the right brain.

After he was discharged from hospital he started physiotherapy, which continued until he was 7 months old. From then he had 'Doman Delacato' method of therapy, 6 days a week for 6 months then 5 days a week for 15 months. His health and sight were improved, and his hearing was very good. His eyes were slightly longsighted. He looked at more things around him, and his concentration was getting better. He started to take weight on his feet. Six months before acupressure treatment he knew where to place his feet when standing and was walking with two hands support. His back and neck continued to get stronger and straighter. He liked to have books read to him and took great interest in the pictures.

At 14 weeks of age he was being given 8 ml of phenobarbitone, decreased at 15 months to 0.5 ml per week for 16 weeks. He then started teething accompanied by slight fitting, so his parents put him back on 5 ml to control it. When he finished teething his mother was to wean him off the drug over 10 weeks.

From May 1989 he received acupressure treatment carried out daily 5 times weekly until July 1989, 52 times in total.

• **Management for speech problems**
The patient received a routine manipulation described below.

1. Pressing the following points 5 to 6 times for one treatment:

• Chuigen (MA point) (see Fig. 3.66).
• Pinching point Dicang (S4) on both sides (see Fig. 3.70).
• Pressing point Yamen (DU15) (see Fig. 3.72).

2. Massage the submandibular region on both sides 20 times for each treatment.

3. Massage along the both sides of laryngeal region 20 times for each treatment.

4. Massage using the thumb and index finger on the hyoid bone 20 times.

• **Management for shoulder problems**
The patient had some limitation of motion in both shoulder joints. The manipulation was the same as described in Chapter 3 (see Figs 3.3, 3.4, 3.5 and 3.6). Do each manipulation 20 times for one treatment.

• **Management for both hip joints**
Clinical examination showed that abduction of the hip joints was limited, and internal rotation was limited on both sides. The 4-form test of legs in prone position was positive in both sides. In the supine position with full extension at the knee joint, the lower limb could

be flexed passively at the hip joint to 45°. (The normal range is 90° or more.) Routine manipulative technique as described in Chapter 3 (see Figs 3.16, 3.17, 3.19 and 3.21) was used. Each manipulation was performed 20 times in a treatment. Results of treatment are shown in Table 6.1.

Table 6.1 Results of treatment

Before treatment	After treatment
1. Mental condition Reactive state slow. Could be vague. Not really 100% aware	Awareness increased. Understands better - likes tickling games. Wants to play - he can understand some orders, he gets angry sometimes, and upset
2. Sat up with rounded back. He had to roll on to his stomach then arched his back to sit up	Able to sit up from a lying position on his back leaning on one elbow. Now sits up with remarkably straight back
3. Unable to stand	After 1 week able to stand against the wall for approximately 1 minute. After 10 weeks able to stand for 10 to 15 minutes. Difficult to keep standing still. Wants to walk
4. Walking. He knew where to place his feet if both hands held above his head	He can now walk slowly holding one hand. Slightly 'wobbly' but balance improving
5. Fits have been decreasing for a long time. On 5 ml phenobarbitone	Still has the same fits, that is 1 half-minute fit every morning or every second morning. On 4 ml phenobarbitone
6. Speech. Could say 'dad-dad', 'mum-mum', 'ba-ba' and had 'intonation' in what sounded like a sentence to him	'Babbles' now with more meaning to the sounds. Shrieks happily - babbles more; happier to do so

The patient, was a retired nurse, and single. Her first visit on 20 May 1989 was for a clinical assessment. Her history included an intracranial haemorrhagic stroke and subdural haematoma while visiting interstate, resulting in quadriplegia, dysphasia, and dizziness for the previous 12 months.

Her cerebrovascular accident had occurred very suddenly 12 months previously with symptoms suggestive of food poisoning. Subsequently she became unconscious and was transferred to a metropolitan hospital. A CT scan revealed a cerebellar haemorrhage, and the presence of a subdural haematoma which was aspirated through a burr hole in the right occipitoparietal region. After the operation she remained in a coma for approximately 6 weeks.

She remained in the hospital for about 5 months until she was well enough to return home for rehabilitation. After that, instead of progressing, she got worse: she imagined things, her balance and walking regressed, she lost her appetite and refused to eat, she became depressed and was rude to those working with her and did not want to continue rehabilitation. However she remained in the rehabilitation centre for about 4 months, where they tried to teach her to walk, improve her speech, and feed herself.

• Clinical examination

The patient came into the consulting room with the support of two people. She had a scanning dysarthric speech of moderate severity, and there was some slight hoarseness of her voice as well. She had slow pursuit movements of the eyes, and she had some vertical nystagmus on looking up, and a few beats of horizontal nystagmus on looking to either side. There was a left facial asymmetry around the mouth and salivation especially when she spoke. The remainder of the cranial nerve examination was unremarkable. Her blood pressure was 130/85 mmHg.

In the periphery, testing of sensation was intact to all modalities. She had some reeling motion of the head and trunk, and there was some slight dysmetria on finger/nose testing, particularly on the left side. Her heel/shin testing also demonstrated dysmetria and moderate ataxia, more marked on the left than the right. She walked with a narrow base, and required the support of two people to remain upright. She tended to fall in any direction. She had some slight resistance to passive movement throughout in the lower limbs, but the resistance to passive movement was normal in the upper limbs. The reflexes were (+++) throughout in both the upper and lower limbs indicating that the reflexes were increased. There was no muscle wasting or weakness, which suggested the physiotherapy she had received for a few months after the acute phase was beneficial.

Clinical impression: this patient certainly had had a severe intracranial haemorrhage and the presence of subdural haematoma post-operation for 12 months. The problems were imbalance in posture control, dizziness, visual problems, communication problems and the original cerebrovascular problem.

• **Acupressure treatment**

The treatment described below was carried out every other day.

1. Pressing 6 points for visual problems 5 or 6 times for each treatment (see Figs 2.1, 2.2 and 2.3):

- Jingming (R1)
- Yuyao (Extra 3)
- Chengqi (S1)
- Sizhukong (SJ 23)
- Fengchi (G20)
- Naokong (G19)

2. Massage along the frontal, and occiptal regions 4 or 5 times each treatment.

3. Treatment of facial paralysis (see Ch. 3).

4. Management for drooling see (see Ch. 3).

5. Speech problems (see Ch. 3).

6. Shoulder, arm, hand, and lower limb problems. These were treated by percussion and routine orthopaedic manipulations: the four shoulder movements; supination of the forearms; flexion, extension, and slight rotation of the hip joints; flexion and extension of the knee joints, upward, downward and rotatory movements of the patellas, dorsal and plantar flexions of the ankle joints, and inversion and eversion movements of the the feet.

7. Walking exercises with the support of a frame to avoid falls.

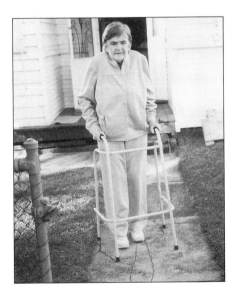

Fig. 6.3 Before treatment standing with the support of a frame

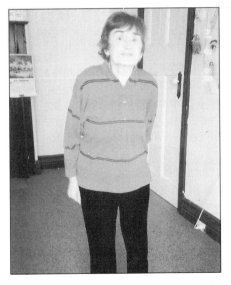

Fig. 6.4 After treatment, the patient stands independently

• Oral administration of Chinese herbs

The patient had a hot temperament, imagining things. She felt dry. Her tongue was dark red in colour, but not furred, indicating intense heat. She had blood stasis due to stagnation of Vital Energy, caused by deficiency of respiration and blood circulation.

A compound prescription containing the ingredients given below was used for herbal treatment of her condition.

• Herbal prescription

Cinnabaris	朱砂	5 g
Radix polygala tenuifolia	遠志	10 g
Semen ziziphi spinosal	棗仁	10 g

For relief of anxiety and to subdue endogenous wind caused by sedatives.

Radix ledebouriellae	防風	15 g
Periostracum cicadue	蟬衣	3 g
Radix condonopsis pilosulae	黨參	15 g
Radix angelical sinensis	當歸	12 g
Radix salviae miltiorrhizae	丹參	15 g
Radix paeoniae rubra	赤芍	12 g

To subdue endogenous wind, reinforce vital energy and invigorate blood circulation.

Radix ophiopogonis	麥冬	12 g
Fructus mume	酸梅	12 g

To promote secretion of body fluid and quench thirst.

Preparation of the herbal mixture

Mix and pour the ingredients into a small pot and then add cold water until the surface of water is 3 cm above the herbs. Boil for 25 minutes. Remove about 60 ml of the fluid and add enough cold water to cover the herbs as before and boil again for 25 minutes. Remove a further 60 ml of the fluid and mix it with the first 60 ml extracted.

The dosage for administration is 30 ml four times daily, half an hour after meals. Each course should be for 40 days, with an interval of 3 weeks before the next course of 40 days.

Side effects

Sometimes there is nausea, with slight abdominal fullness and discomfort and one or two soft stools within 24 hours. If the symptoms appear, discontinue the herbal treatment for 1 to 2 days.

• **Results of treatment**

The patient had acupressure therapy 45 times and oral administration of Chinese herbal decoction for 20 days. Her symptoms and signs were improved, and the clinical changes were as shown in Table 6.2.

Table 6.2 Results of treatment

Before treatment	After treatment
1. Appetite poor	Better
2. Imagining things	Improved
3. Balance	Improved
4. Drooling	Ceased after 12 sessions
5. Vision	Improved
6. Speech	Improved. Clearer
7. Shoulder motions. Elevation of arms to 150° Unable to touch opposite ear. Unable to touch spine with thumbs	Elevation of arms to 170° Able to touch opposite ears. Able to touch spine with thumbs
8. Forearm supination limited in both sides	Improved in both sides
9. Stood with frame support	Stands independently
10. Walked with frame support	Walks without support
11. Motions in both hip joints. Internal rotation limited External rotation limited Stretch and elevation of legs limited	Internal rotation improved External rotation improved Stretch and elevation of legs normal
12. Dark red tongue. No fur	Better
13. Dry and thirsty	Improved

CASE HISTORY — Male, aged 64 years

Date of first visit May 1989. Chief complaint: right sided hemiplegia with functional disturbance for 3 years.

Present illness: This gentleman originally presented with an episode of sudden transitory partial blind areas in the field of vision on the right side in March 1986. Subsequently he was admitted to the haematology department of a metropolitan hospital with a history of lesion of the right fifth cranial nerve over a period of 14 hours, fluctuating upper motor weakness in the right limbs, and dysarthria. He had an elevated haemoglobin count and underwent acute haemodilution. He had good resolution of his neurological deficit and no major large vessel obstruction could be identified. The red cell mass and plasma volume studies after venesection were normal, but on calculation of red cell mass from the total volume of blood removed, there was probably a significant increase. His B^{12} binding level was also elevated and folate was reduced. The bone marrow was hypercellular with a relative increase in the erythroid precursors. Myeloid cells and megakaryocytes were normal. The marrow reticulum was not increased. A firm diagnosis of polycythaemia rubra vera was not made and the patient was discharged for follow-up.

On 2 July 1986 the patient was again admitted to hospital for a temporal artery biopsy. The biopsy report was normal. He received treatment of prednisolone 50 mg/day and cyclophosphamide 100mg/day. He had many reactive changes in his haematology with neutrophilia, eosinophilia, thrombocytosis and an elevated ESR. There were also significant changes on haemorrheology. The possibility that this patient may have had underlying myeloproliferative disease was considered but could not be confirmed by bone marrow examination or other haematological investigations.

• Acupressure treatment

On 3 May 1989 the patient commenced acupressure therapy for right sided hemiplegia which he had had for 3 years. The treatment was carried out once every day for 4 weeks, and 3 times weekly for 1 month, giving a total of 32 treatments. The treatment for the management of facial paralysis and the speech problems followed the method described in Chapter 3.

• Right arm

1. General percussion along the first, second, fourth, fifth and sixth stimulation lines for about 10 minutes.

2. Pressing the following points about 10 times on each point for one treatment:

- Jianyu (LI 15). Location: antero-inferior to the acromion, on the upper portion of the Deltoid muscle. When the arm is in full abduction, the point is in the depression appearing at the anterior border of the arm (see Fig. 2.1).
- Bingfeng (SI12). Location: in the centre of the suprascapular fossa, directly above Tianzong (SI11); when the arm is lifted, the point is at the site of the depression (see Fig. 2.2).

- Tianzong (SI11). Location: in the infrascapular fossa, at the junction of the upper and middle third of a vertical line between the lower border of the scapular spine and the inferior angle of the scapula (see Fig. 2.2).
- Zhima (MA point). Location: 5 cm below the axillary line, at the midline of the internal aspect of the arm (see Fig. 2.1).
- Xiabai (LU4). Location: on the front of the arm at side of Biceps brachii muscle (see Fig. 2.1).
- Waiguan (SJ 5). Location: 6 cm above point Yangchi (SJ 4), between the radius and ulna (see Fig. 2.3).
- Neiguan (P6). Location: 6 cm above the transverse flexion crease at the wrist, between the tendons of the Palmaris longus and Flexor carpi radialis muscles (see Fig. 2.1).
- Zhangjian (MA point). Location: 1 cm above the metacarpophalangeal joint, the three Zhangjian points are located in the spaces separating the second and third, the third and fourth, and the fourth and fifth metacarpals (see Fig. 2.2).
- Zhiguanjie (MA point). Location: around the proximal and distal interphalangeal joints of the index, middle, ring and little fingers of the hand (see Fig. 2.1).
- Zhijiagen (MA point). Location: at the nail fold of the 4 fingers and thumb, above the nail roots (see Fig. 2.2).

There was no deformity in the right arm, so that the orthopaedic manipulations were not required.

Functional exercises were done such as making a fist, touching the thumb with the tips of the fingers, picking up small objects, writing words, etc.

• Right lower limb
1. Percussion along the first, second, fourth, sixth and eighth stimulation lines was carried out for the purpose of promoting the blood circulation and improving the nerve conduction in the lower limb.
2. Pressing points such as Huantiao (G30), Yinmen (B37), Weizhong (B40), Chengshan (B57), Genjian (MA point), Biguan (S31), Futu (S32), Zusanli (S36), Fenglong (S40), Jiexi (S41), Zhiguanjie (MA point), Zhijiagen (MA point) (see Figs 2.1, 2.2, and 2.3).
3. Exercises, such as elevation of the leg, dorsiflexion of ankle joint, squatting, walking, etc.

Results of treatment are shown in Table 6.3 on the next page.

Table 6.3 Results of treatment

Before treatment	After treatment
1. Right leg	
Drop foot led to difficulty when walking	Improved. Walk easier
Toes would not always stay outstretched during walking	Improved as above
Toes curled under	Improved
Foot turned inwards	Improved
Knee sometimes weak	Improved. Control increased, both in flexion and extension
Heel numb	Improved
Hamstring muscle itchy at back of leg	Improved. Blood circulation in right leg very good
Right foot was colder than left	Temperature equal in both feet. Heel up/down control good
2. Lower back ache sometimes	Lower back ache disappeared
3. Right arm Hand difficult to control accurately	Right hand function much better, control good
Numbness of the fingers at the tips and also in thumb. Stiffness in proximal and distal interphalangel joints. Sometimes this sensation extended to elbow joint.	Sensation of fingers and thumb recovered, and movements in interphalageal joints in normal range. Also ability to pick up small objects with fingers greatly improved
4. During walking there was fatigue from forearm to back of neck	In patient's own words, 'I feel 90% recovered'
5. Face and head Difficulty turning head fully to left or right	Improved. More flexible
Right side of face numb from cheek, nose to mouth	Face sensation recovered. Slight improvement
Difficulty chewing on right side	Slight improvement
Speaking difficult sometimes	Better after treatment
Words with many vowels difficult to pronounce	Very much improved
Intensity of facial numbness varied from time to time	Much improved
Muscular restriction in throat appeared sometimes to cause coughing	Improved. (This symptom may be due to muscle spasm)
Consumption of small amounts of alcohol appeared to cause slight headache	Recommended that the patient did not drink any alcohol
6. General condition	In the patient's own words: 'My feeling of good health is the best for 5 years'

• Patient's questions

This patient asked a number of questions related to his treatment that are of general interest, and they are discussed below.

The patient asked whether cortisone could cause muscle deterioration. The effects of cortisone treatment are well established. Adverse reactions include muscular weakness as an occasional side effect of most corticosteroids, particularly when they are taken in large doses.

In my experience the use of cortisones over a long period of time, a few years' use, causes severe complications involving weakness of the muscles. At a conference on the treatment of rheumatoid arthritis, held in Beijing in 1983, a paper was presented summarizing the results of treatment of 150 patients from 8 different hospitals across China. The report indicated that the prolonged use of prednisone caused ischaemic necrosis of the head of the femur. It was also found that all patients treated with prednisone had this complication, not only the patients with rheumatoid arthritis.

The patient asked whether he should stop the cortisone treatment. I recommended that after consultation with his clinical haematologist he stop taking cortisone.

He also asked whether I considered that his present conditon would be maintained. I answered that it would improve if he had a regular daily life and did home exercises. He should take care to sleep well, to avoid getting overtired, angry or upset, and to dress warmly during winter to prevent catching cold. He should take care against falls or any damage. Alcohol would be also very bad for his condition. If such a lifestyle were maintained, then he should retain his improved level of condition. If not, then his condition might deteriorate.

The people of China have a saying that in the treatment of disease, 30% is the doctor's work and 70% is the patient's work. This means taking rest and nourishment to regain health. This saying summarizes the experience of the Chinese people over thousands of years.

QUESTIONS AND ANSWERS

Q. What improvement can be expected in a child with cerebral birth injury after the 3 months of acupressure therapy?

A. It is impossible to give a specific prediction because each child responds according to his or her original level of incapacity, therefore each will be different. The clinical results of this therapy are generally good and we are confident that it will help most patients.

Q. Can the therapy also be used for CVA patients or patients with brain damage associated with head injury?

A. Yes, the same therapy is useful for these types of patient.

Q. What improvement can be expected in a CVA patient or a brain injury patient after 3 months of acupressure therapy?

A. As with children each adult patient's response to therapy varies, however clinical results are generally also good with these patients.

Q. What factors are different between patients
    with cerebral birth injury and adult CVA or
    injury patients?

A. The developmental factor is absent in
    adults. Thus an adult CVA patient has to
    recover a capacity, such as speech, that he
    or she has already learned, whereas a child
    may yet have to develop the capacity.

Q. When, or at what age, is the treatment no
    longer useful with children?

A. The younger the child, the better the
    results. The treatment is less effective in
    children over the age of 10. However, we
    have treated a few patients aged 11 to 16,
    whose condition has improved.

Q. Should every patient be recommended an
    individual treatment programme (i.e., what
    points, type of percussion or manipulation
    and the frequency)?

A. Yes, a programme tailored to suit each
    individual is an integral part of the therapy.

Q. Why is the treatment over in 12 weeks?
    What is the reason for this length of time?

A. According to our clinical experience, this is
    the average time required, however some
    patients may require less and others more,
    in some cases up to 6 months.

Q.   Once an improvement has been achieved, will it be permanent or will it regress?

A.   The improvements gained can be maintained by the patient making use of the improved abilities (if necessary with the parent's help).

Q.   How can parents best maintain and or improve further on the level reached?

A.   By continuing with the therapy and making sure the child is made to use the improved faculties.

Q.   Are parents expected to continue the treatment themselves at home, and for how long?

A.   Yes, they are, and they should continue until the child is near normal or the recovery is complete.

Q.   Are parents taught how to continue the therapy with their children?

A.   Every parent can readily be shown how to treat his or her own child. The teaching should be an integral part of the therapy.

Q.   How can one tell that the therapy is no longer beneficial and that it should cease?

A.   When the recovery is complete, stop. If there is no progress after a long period of treatment, stop for 3 or 4 weeks then start again.

Q. Is there a need for reassessment and changes in the therapy programme?

A. Yes, there should be a routine assessment.

Q. Should children continue wearing their callipers, AFOs (ankle-foot orthoses), etc., while having treatment (and after)?

A. Yes, as long as these aids are absolutely necessary to the children, but it is essential that they make use of any new ability that they have gained and not become lazy with the use of mechanical help. Exercise your own judgement.

Q. Does the treatment improve intellectual capacity?

A. Yes, but the improvement is small. Children with mental retardation require special exercises.

Q. While undergoing acupressure therapy should other forms of treatment (e.g., physiotherapy) be discontinued or are the treatments complementary to one another?

A. Combining with orthopaedic manipulation is helpful; the important aspect is that the therapy must be applied for specific purposes following a diagnosis.

Q.   What exercises/techniques are most beneficial for gaining walking skills?

A.   With each child it is necessary to address the particular affected areas which influence his or her walking (i.e., limitation of joint movement, contraction and spasm of the affected joint, lesion or poor development of the joint).

Q.   I understand that percussion is aimed at relaxing the muscles to allow better movement, and I understand the need for relaxation of muscles with high tone. How does the same technique apply to muscles with low or fluctuating tone? How does the technique vary for one or the other?

A.   The therapy involves techniques for both high and low muscle tone. Percussion can both reduce muscle spasm and increase muscle tone depending on the strength and intensity of the percussion. Pressing and stretching techniques are also applied as needed and the points are different.

Q.   Will the treatment reduce scoliosis in children, and if it does, will the improvement be permanent?

A.   The effectiveness of our treatment on scoliosis is limited, but an improved muscle tone will minimise scoliosis.

Q. Is there an acupressure treatment for epilepsy?

A. Epilepsy is generally successfully treated by the combination of antiepileptic drugs and pressing antiepileptic points.

Q. How can acupressure therapy help fits (myclonic jerks)?

A. It is necessary to identify the causes first (i.e., muscle spasm, or irregularity of movement) and address the treatment to these.

Q. What will happen if a child has not shown any or little improvement at the end of the 3 months of therapy?

A. This does not mean that there cannot be improvement. I recommend giving the child a rest for 1 month and then starting again.

POSTSCRIPT

I worked for about 25 years as an orthopaedic surgeon before undergoing training in traditional Chinese medicine. Whenever I recall my work as a surgeon with cerebral palsied patients, my mind is in a turmoil, because I could not do more for them. Only a few small operations can be done in highly selected cases. I was unable to treat multiple neurological deficits and functional disturbances. I could only give a prescription for drugs and ask patients to do some exercises at home. I understood that the patients could do little at home. I had come to the end of my tether. However, after I trained in traditional Chinese medicine, especially acupressure therapy, and used this method in the treatment of cerebral palsied children and some adult patients, I have obtained good results. Since I changed to this special method, I have also been able to do more for patients with brain problems.

We are grateful for the special action of acupressure therapy which both relaxes spasticity and increases muscle tone. The application of this ancient method has been newly developed as a technique in clinical practice for treating difficult and complicated cases. This book has covered in particular the sequelae of cerebral birth injury, brain injury and cerebrovascular accident, and reviews the benefits, including curative effects, which may be achieved through acupressure therapy.

The manipulative technique called acupressure looks very easy, and indeed we often teach the parents to treat their own children at home.

However, when studied more deeply there are some practical difficulties. One misconception is that acupressure therapy technique can be separated from the needs of the patients. It is essential that before treatment one takes the case history, makes the proper diagnosis, and plans for a treatment based on the overall analysis of the illness and the patient's condition.

If one wants to make a proper diagnosis and ensure good treatment for patients with problems of the central nervous system, especially in the above described three groups of patients, it is essential to have the knowledge of acupressure therapy, Chinese acupuncture, neurology, anatomy, orthopaedics, physiotherapy, paediatrics, cardiovascular disease, and haemotology, etc. The clinical work is hard. One course of treatment often needs 3 months or longer, so there must be indomitable will, and unshakable and full confidence by therapists, parents, and even the very young patients. The curative effect gradually appears in the process of treatment. Another point that the parents or patients should understand, is that the work is not finished or stopped after 3 months clinical treatment. Patients and parents need to continue some of the manipulations and exercises at home for a long time. Some neurological deficits or deformities cannot be completely corrected or recovered, so expectations that are too high can disappoint parents and patients.

We continue to study and perfect this technique and we hope to be able to share the advantages of acupressure therapy with doctors, therapists, parents and patients throughout the world. Acupressure therapy techniques cover new ground in the treatment of cerebral birth injury, brain damage due to injury or cerebrovascular accident. The potential of this technique has not yet been fully realized, even in China, where research in this area has shown evidence of improved blood circulation (both cardiovascular and peripheral) improved nerve conduction and an effect on the somatosensory evocative potential.

We hope that this book will contribute to world recognition of the potential of these techniques and that further research will thus be encouraged.

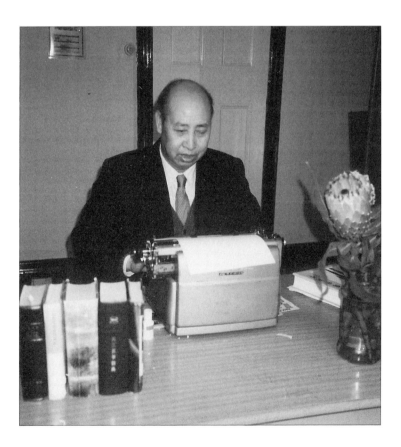

REFERENCES

Cheng Xin-nong 1987 Chinese acupuncture and moxibustion. Foreign Languages Press, Beijing

Guo Guang-wen et al 1986 Colour atlas of human anatomy. The People's Health Publishing House, Beijing

Jennett B, Teasdale G 1981 Management of head injuries. F A Davis, Philadelphia (Contemporary Neurology, Vol 20)

Jia Li-hui 1986 Pointing therapy: a Chinese traditional therapeutic skill. Shandong Science and Technology Press, Shandong

Jin Shi-ying et al 1984 An atlas of acupuncture points, 4th edn. The People's Health Publishing House, Beijing

Kaplan P E, Cerulo L J (eds) 1986 Stroke rehabilitation. Butterworth, Stoneham

Levitt, S 1982 Treatment of cerebral palsy and motor delay, 2nd edn. Blackwell Scientific, Oxford

Strang I, Jennett B, Macmillan R 1978 Head injuries in accident and emergency departments at Scottish hospitals. Injury 10(2): 154-159

Sutin J A 1986 Clinical presentation of stroke syndromes. In: Kaplan P E, Cerulo L J (eds) Stroke rehabilitation. Butterworth, Stoneham

Wang Zhao-pu 1988 Sequelae of cerebral birth injury in infants treated by acupressure. Journal of Traditional Chinese Medicine 8(1): 19-22

INDEX